BOSH!
MEAT

When using kitchen appliances please always follow the manufacturer's instructions.

HQ
An imprint of HarperCollins*Publishers* Ltd
1 London Bridge Street
London SE1 9GF

www.harpercollins.co.uk

HarperCollins*Publishers*
Macken House, 39/40 Mayor Street Upper,
Dublin 1, D01 C9W8, Ireland

10 9 8 7 6 5 4 3 2 1

First published in Great Britain by
HQ, an imprint of HarperCollins*Publishers* Ltd 2023

ISBN: 978-0-00-842073-4
Exclusive Editon ISBN:978-0-00-863948-8

This book is produced from independently certified FSC™
paper to ensure responsible forest management.
For more information visit:
www.harpercollins.co.uk/green

Food photography: Lizzie Mayson
Lifestyle photography: Nicky Johnston
Food styling: Eleanor Mulligan
Prop styling: Louie Waller
Project Editor: Laura Nickoll
Senior Editor: Nira Begum
Book Design: Studio Polka
Senior Production Controller: Halema Begum

Printed and bound in Italy by Rotolito S.p.A.

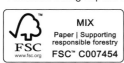

MIX
Paper | Supporting
responsible forestry
FSC™ C007454

DELICIOUS. HEARTY. PLANT-BASED.

BOSH!
MEAT

HENRY FIRTH & IAN THEASBY

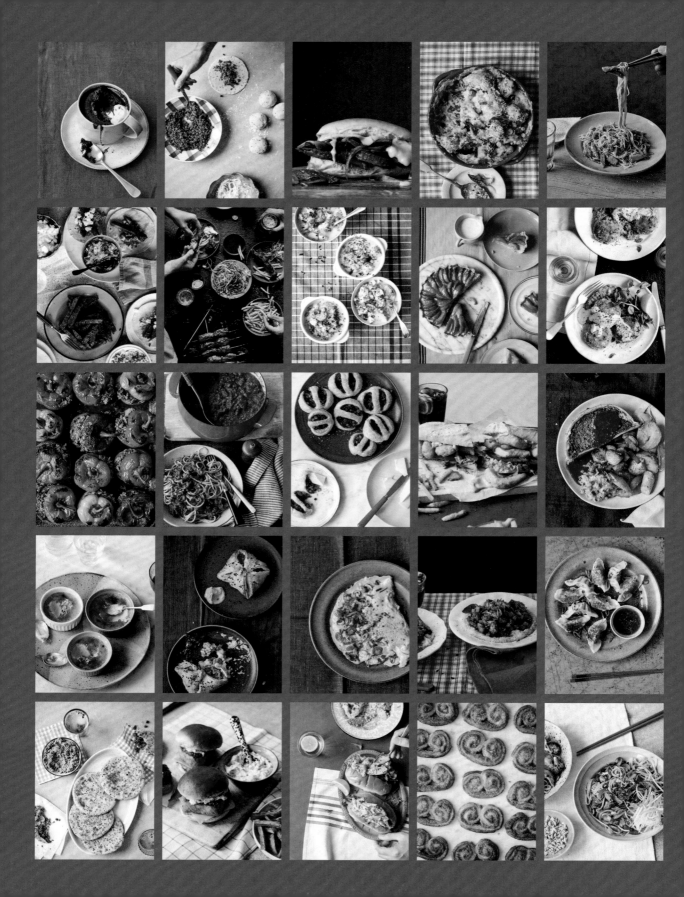

WELCOME
6

THE FUTURE OF MEAT IS PLANTS
10

HOW TO MAKE MEAT
24

POULTRY
42

BEEF
76

PORK
108

LAMB
136

SEAFOOD
168

CHEESE
200

DESSERTS
220

INDEX
246

CONVERSION CHARTS
254

ACKNOWLEDGEMENTS
255

WELCOME

Hello, and welcome to our best book yet! In the last five years we've written six books, selling over a million copies, and in that time we've watched the world change. With more and more delicious food available in stores than ever, it's finally our time to conquer meat. At last, we can bring you the tastiest food on Planet Earth, all made entirely from plants.

There's a food revolution happening right now, there's a new way of cooking. We're going to create all your favourite meaty dishes, but without using any animals whatsoever.

It's magical. It's inspiring. This way of thinking about food is at the forefront of culinary innovation. We've been eating animals for millennia, but only in the last five years has it become possible to cook absolutely any dish using plant-based ingredients. Wonderful!

When we started creating recipes, plant-based dishes were all made of, well, just fruits and vegetables. But this has evolved, and geniuses have been innovating, and now, it's as easy as pie to enjoy burgers, steaks, sausages, wings and more, created entirely from plants.

Why meat, you may ask? Well, we are, and always have been, meat-lovers at heart. We love those complex, savoury, meaty flavours. There's nothing wrong with liking the taste of chicken! But what we don't love is the other stuff that comes with it: the way animals are treated, and the way meat is produced commercially can be irresponsible and often feels medieval. We don't want any part of that! And we care deeply about the planet too, preserving it for future generations.

We're going to show you just how tasty plants can be, and how dishes can look, feel and taste just like meat. Learn how to cook brilliant meals that will satisfy, impress and delight, all using products that are easy to find on supermarket shelves.

From big show-stopping dishes, super-simple quick dinners and great ideas for lunches to phenomenal sweet treats and much, much more, this book has it all. Whether you choose to buy plant-based meat or make it yourself at home, we've got you covered.

So, if you're a meat-eater looking to eat less, or you're a veggie or a flexi, this book is for you. And a uniquely tasty world of flavour awaits!

Big love,

Henry and Ian x BOSH!

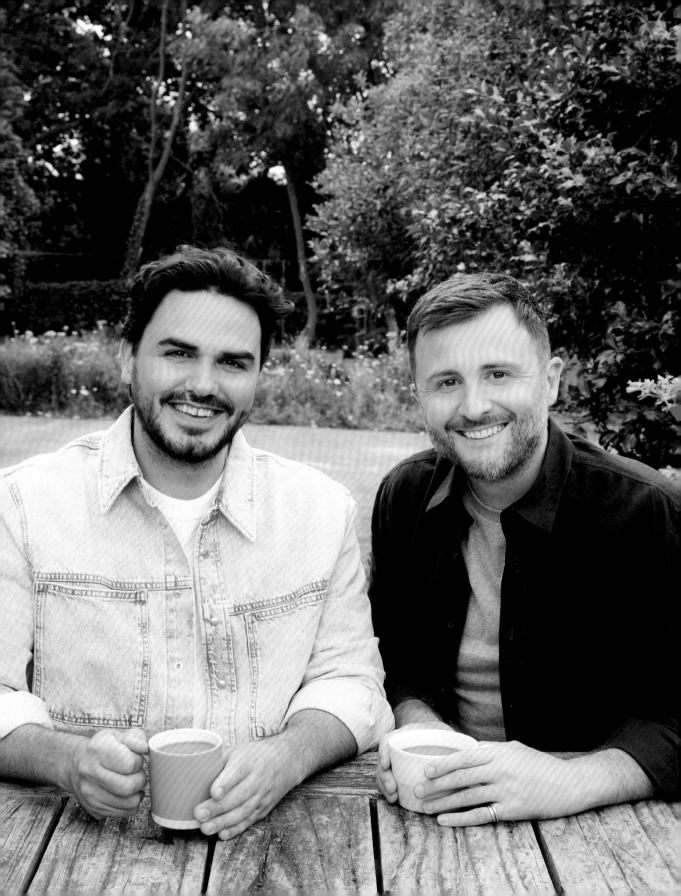

IN THIS BOOK

What is plant-based meat?

Plant-based meat is meat that is derived directly from plants rather than animals. Often, it will contain protein from beans (soy or pea), wheat or potato, vegetables and natural added flavours. And sometimes, a plant meat is just a combination of vegetables, nuts, grains or other plants that tastes or looks just like meat, when cooked in the right way! It can be bought in shops or made at home (see pages 26–41) and is intended to recreate the flavour and texture of animal meat. Plant-based meat is typically better for the planet and can be great for you too.

A meaty book made from plants

This book is divided into meaty chapters, so you can search for recipes by flavour. If you're looking for a red meat flavour, or a vibrant chicken-y dish, simply head to the relevant chapter. You'll also find cheese dishes and desserts that are so good you simply won't believe they're made from plants.

Plant meats and meaty plants

These recipes deliver a full meaty punch, are packed with flavour and protein and taste delicious. Discover wonderful ways to create dishes from the plant-based meats and recipes that celebrate the vegetable, using ingredients like mushrooms and jackfruit to deliver that familiar protein texture.

All the flavour, all the texture

We'll show you how to layer ingredients like soy sauce, Marmite or tomato purée to create a rich savoury flavour. And we'll show you how to create meaty textures using different ingredients with different properties, cooking and seasoning them perfectly.

Shop-bought (or home-made)

Everyone has busy lives, so we've made sure we focus on ingredients you can easily buy. This is the ultimate guide to cooking with those plant-based ingredients you can now find in most supermarkets and local stores! But if you are the kind of home cook who likes to spend time in the kitchen, you can also create your own beef, chicken, milk, cheese and more.

Incredible colours and flavours

Flick through the book to see the colours of the rainbow across our dishes! Colour is such an important part of healthy eating, as your body naturally craves plant nutrients, so we'll help you stay healthy by eating plants of all varieties while enjoying incredibly satisfying meals.

Food for every day and every occasion

You'll find weeknight recipes, showstopping dinners and more involved feasts, quick food, slow food, sandwiches, dinners, lunches and desserts. You'll find cooking techniques that are simple, and some that are more complex. You'll find unique creations and reinvented restaurant classics. And you'll find favourite dishes from around the world, from a huge variety of different cuisines. We sincerely hope this will be your new favourite cookbook!

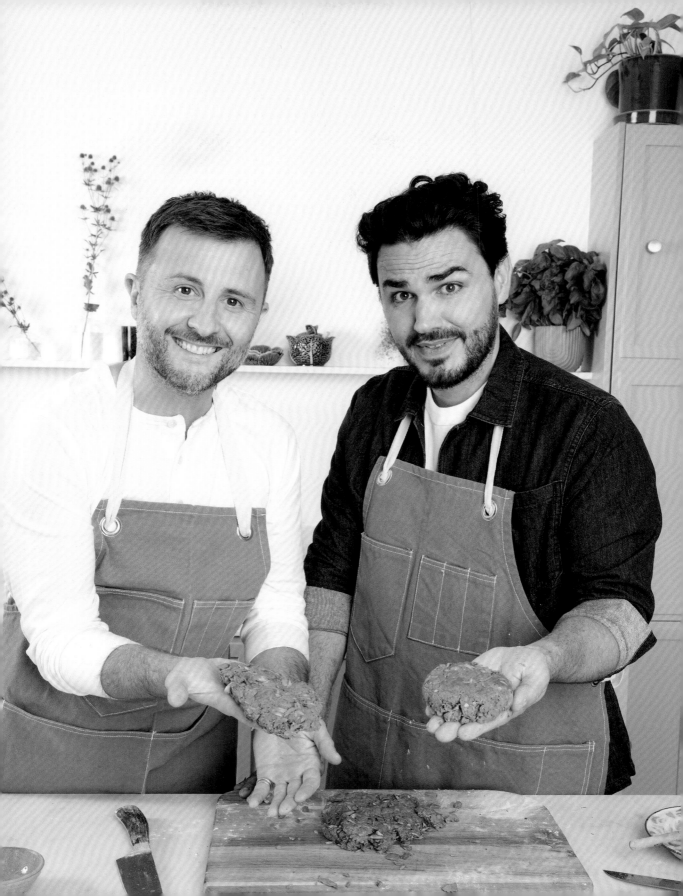

THE FUTURE OF MEAT IS PLANTS

WELCOME TO A NEW WAY OF THINKING ABOUT MEAT
Historically, meat was incredibly important for the survival of humanity. Eating animals provided a powerful source of nutrients and stored energy. It's no wonder the practice of eating meat is so ingrained in our traditions.

OUR TASTES ARE EVOLVING
We're becoming conscious of the impact we're having on the world. It's no longer just the flavour that matters, we now want foods that make a positive impact, and processes such as 'fair trade' and 'organic' explaining the origin and journey of a product. We think about our choices, what's good for us and the planet and we're creating new, better food systems. This means we can still enjoy the foods we love, but it's possible for those foods to be plant-based.

ENERGY FROM THE SUN
Plants turn solar energy into calories we can eat. They take energy from sunlight, mix it with water and grow. When we eat plants, we harness that energy from the sun in the form of calories. This is a very efficient process because it's clean, renewable food energy for our bodies. You might even say that eating a plant burger is comparable to driving an electric car: it's a great experience first and foremost, but it also feels modern, fresh and cool. It's logical and responsible. By comparison, a burger made from animals uses more resources and creates significantly more waste. Animal agriculture uses a disproportionately large amount of land and water and is responsible for emitting far more greenhouse gas emissions than plant-based food systems. It's simply a less efficient way of getting energy from food.

THIS IS THE START OF A NEW ERA
More companies than ever before are turning their focus to plant-based meats, so things can only get better. What a time to be alive!

HOW IS IT GOOD FOR ME AND FOR THE PLANET?
As a general rule, and according to studies by Oxford University, Harvard and Future Foods, plant-based alternatives are better for the environment and for human health than their animal-based counterparts. Plant-based products tend to contain better nutritional profiles compared to animal products*. Studies have also shown it's more efficient to make food from plants than from animals. Plant-based products cause lower levels of greenhouse gas emissions, they generally need less land and water, and are less polluting. And as plant-based food technologies improve, plant meats will become even better and more energy-efficient to produce.

—

*Sources: the UK's nutrient profiling model and bath.ac.uk/announcements/plant-based-meat-healthier-and-more-sustainable-than-animal-products-new-study

PLANT MEAT CHEAT SHEET

A FOOD REVOLUTION

We're at the forefront of this food revolution. New products, ingredients and cooking techniques for plant-based meats are being created every month. There is a smorgasbord of options out there.

A HEALTH-FOCUSED ALTERNATIVE

A healthy diet involves a balanced intake of many elements, including protein. The human body needs protein to help repair, maintain and generate new cells, especially for bones and muscles. Historically, the easy way to get protein into the diet was to eat animal proteins like meat, dairy and eggs. However, plant-based foods can also be rich in protein, including ingredients such as beans, grains, nuts and soy. Now, with the modern development in plant-based meats, it's even easier to get protein into your diet.

IS PLANT MEAT GOOD FOR ME?

Simply put, it depends on what you eat, and how often. There are brands you can buy and ways you can prepare plant meat that are great for you, and plant meats are typically packed with protein, fortified with vitamins, and high in fibre. But, as with all things, you'll find there are brands that use too many chemicals or load their foods with salt or saturated fat. Should you eat bacon every day? Probably not, regardless of whether it's made from plants or animals!

HOW DO I CHOOSE?

We've created a super-simple guide to reading labels, to help you navigate your way through the different plant-meat brands (pages 18–19). Get into the habit of reading labels, so you can find out what's in the foods before you buy them. Try different brands and you'll find your new favourites. Learn about the food you eat, and take charge of your own wellbeing. Learn what you like, what's good for you, and what to avoid. And always talk to a doctor or qualified dietician if you're not sure.

When should I eat it?

It's obviously up to you when to eat plant meat. You might eat it at every meal, or once to a couple of times per week, it's absolutely your call. The good news is, you can swap out animal meat for plant meat in any recipe you like, whether it's from this book or somewhere else. Familiarise yourself with a few brands or try a few techniques to make your own and you'll be able to freestyle any recipe with ease.

What if I'm eating for the gym or on a diet?

Plant meats can work brilliantly to support your gym workouts or diets, even if you're on a keto diet. They are packed with protein and can support muscle building. Just be sure to check in with your trainer, nutritionist or doctor and do your own research.

This chart illustrates the difference in impact that plant-based meat products have on the planet in terms of carbon dioxide emissions compared to animal-based products.

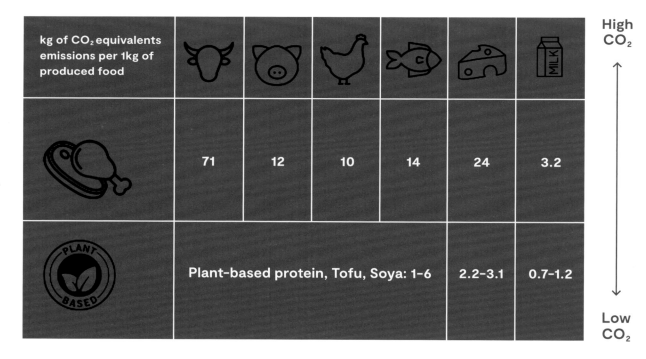

kg of CO_2 equivalents emissions per 1kg of produced food	🐂	🐖	🐔	🐟	🧀	🥛	High CO_2
	71	12	10	14	24	3.2	
	Plant-based protein, Tofu, Soya: 1–6				2.2–3.1	0.7–1.2	Low CO_2

Sources for emissions data: Beef, pork, chicken, pea protein – plantbasednews.org; farmed fish, tofu, milks – ourworldindata.org; cheese vs plant-based cheese – violifefoods.com report by Quantis sustainability consultancy, April 2022; soy – consumerecology.com; seitan – theveganreview.com; plant-based burger substitutes – sciencedirect.com/science/article/pii/S2666833522000612#bib0085

A BRIEF HISTORY OF PLANT MEAT

Ancient wisdom

Meat alternatives seem to have popped up in the last five years, but in reality they've been around a lot longer. Tofu was first mentioned in the book Simple and Exotic by Chinese writer Tao Ku in 995 CE, and apparently seitan was discovered by Buddhist monks almost 1,500 years ago! Obviously, we weren't around then, so we will recount what we've noticed since going plant-based.

2015–2020

Room to grow

In 2015, the only plant-based products in big supermarket fridges were bean burgers and falafel. If you wanted plant-based milk, you'd be drinking soy milk. High-end dark chocolate was the only plant-based confectionary and margarine was the only plant-based dairy alternative. If you were really lucky, you'd find plant-based sausages in the freezer.

2020s

Adoption begins

At the beginning of the 2020s the plant-based offering in supermarkets exploded. Jackfruit, banana blossom, tempeh, tofu, king oyster mushrooms, plant-based sausages, burgers, bacon and chicken joined oat, coconut and hazelnut milks along with a whole host of cookies, doughnuts and cakes. Spreadable plant-based butter and meltable cheese complemented freezers full of plant-based sausages, pizzas, fish fingers, meatballs and ice cream. You can now get almost anything you want in the supermarkets. The last few years have been a period of revolutionary change, but things are only just getting started.

2022+

Systemic change

Plant-based food has become big business. New manufacturing facilities and techniques will produce a higher volume of plant-based meat that will be cheaper and tastier than ever before, leading to a higher rate of sale, taking market share from animal-derived meat. Revenue and marketing budgets will grow. As young, early adopters of plant-based products grow older, they'll impart their plant-based buying habits onto their children which will see the industry transform to a plants-first system with animal-derived products becoming rare and expensive. This might seem like science fiction now, but this can easily become reality. Think about mobile phones today and how they are infinitely more advanced than they were 20 years ago. Imagine what plant-based meat will be like 20 years from now. It really is extremely exciting.

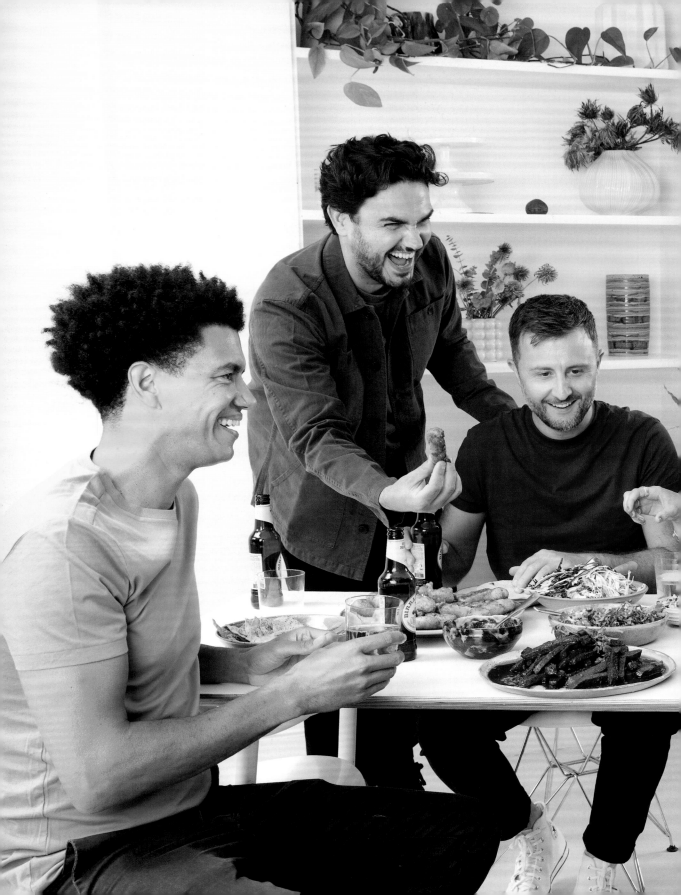

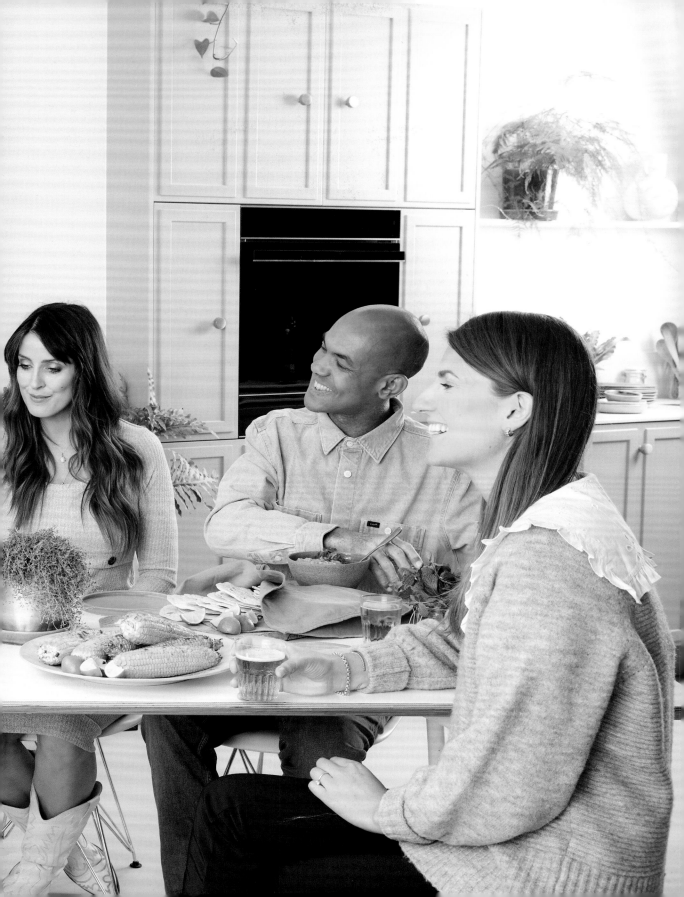

LIVE WELL

We should all be thinking about our health. We firmly believe that paying attention to our nutrition is important in order to live a healthy, abundant life. As you may know, we swear by our 5 Golden Rules. These rules are our pillars we stand by to ensure we eat well and stay healthy. They're a great place to start.

1. The Rainbow Ratio: 50/25/25

Aim to eat roughly 50% fruits and veggies, 25% wholegrains and 25% protein. This ratio will help you achieve a balanced diet.

2. Mix Up Your Plate

Get a wide variety of foods on your plate at every meal. Different colours, textures, ingredients and flavours will not only keep your body happy but your taste buds will be pleased too!

3. Eat Your Greens!

This is an obvious one but it's easy to forget. The more green leafy veg you eat, the better!

4. Aim for 80/20

Simple but super effective; eat healthy food 80% of the time and treat yourself to naughty(ish) food for the remaining 20%.

When it comes to plant-based meat alternatives, the fourth rule of our five golden rules – aim for 80/20 – is the most important. On average, we cook with plant-based meat alternatives a couple of times a week; they're fun to cook with and, when prepared properly, super tasty. However, plant-based meat is processed food; some of the products out there can be high in saturated fat and sodium, with some including artificial colouring, preservatives and flavouring in their ingredient lists. We think that, like anything in life, finding balance is important. In this book we've got a really nice balance of recipes that use plant-based meat alternatives and recipes that use meaty vegetables.

5. Get Your Vits In

An easy way to make sure you're getting your vitamins in is to take a multivitamin every day. This isn't just for people who eat exclusively plant-based, it's for everyone! (You know it makes sense.)

HOW TO READ LABELS

It can be a minefield finding your way around the supermarket and finding the right products to eat! Reading labels is the most important thing, so you understand what is in the products you are buying. For us, there are some ingredients we are fine with and some we eat less of or avoid altogether.

As a general rule, we try to eat as many whole foods, plants, vegetables, fruits, nuts, seeds as possible, but we also welcome the new plant meats arriving in stores.

There are plenty of compounds that sound scary but actually aren't when you look into them. Some things such as Methylcellulose gets a bad name, but it's in fact just a thickener or emulsifier found in most foods – sauces, dressings, meat, plant meat, ice creams, breads, cakes and chocolate.

Plant foods are new, and the space is evolving, so it can be hard to keep up. **On the next two pages** are lists of ingredients that can be commonly found in plant foods, which we've sorted into what we eat lots of, some of, less of and what we avoid.

As always, do your own research, make your own decisions and seek advice if you need to. We're chefs, not nutritionists. This shows you how we like to make our decisions.

EAT MOSTLY

We make a point of seeking out plant foods made with these wholesome ingredients

PLANTS

- **Lentils** – source of fibre and micronutrients
- **Mushrooms** – antioxidant and antimicrobial properties
- **Nuts and seeds** – source of healthy fats, fibre, vitamins and minerals
- **Beans and legumes** – source of protein and micronutrients
- **Jackfruit** – source of antioxidants and fibre; enhances immunity, digestion and heart health
- **Natto** (fermented soybeans) – like tofu, but extra fermentation adds probiotics. Higher concentration of nutrients and protein. Enhances digestive and heart health
- **Soy, almond, coconut milk** – naturally extracted from base ingredients
- **Seitan** – high in protein, but shop versions often high in preservatives and salt
- **Tempeh** – similar fermentation process to natto (above); can help lower cholesterol and is less processed than tofu. Still requires preservatives
- **Tofu** – great source of protective antioxidants

NATURAL FLAVOURINGS AND COLOURINGS

- Fruit/veg concentrates, herbs and spices, nutritional yeast

EAT SOME

These processed products often appear in plant foods and aren't intrinsically bad for you if consumed in moderation

PROTEINS

- **Pea protein • Soya protein • Rice protein • Wheat protein • Chickpea protein • Mycoprotein**

FLAVOURINGS

- **Natural flavourings • Yeast flavourings • Herbs and spices • Salt**

FATS

- **Coconut oil • Vegetable oil • Sunflower oil • Shea oil • Rapeseed oil**

BINDERS

- **Bamboo fibre • Potato fibre / starch • Pea fibre**

EAT LESS

Check labels for these highly processed ingredients and consider those foods as an occasional treat

FILLERS

- **Maltodextrin** – a highly processed vegetable starch, similar to corn syrup
- **Processed gums** such as gellan gum, E418

PRESERVATIVES

- **Sodium metabisulfite**, E223
- **Diphosphates**, E450
- **Calcium acetate**, E263

In general, we watch out for the positioning of processed ingredients on the food ingredient label: the lower down the better, as that means there's little of it.

AVOID

Steer clear of plant foods containing these ingredients if you can – they are not necessary for making delicious plant foods and a high intake is generally considered bad for your health

FOODS THAT ARE HIGH IN:

- **Salt:** may be listed as sodium chloride, potassium chloride or calcium chloride
- **Saturated fat** and/or calories
- **Sugar and/or high fructose** corn syrup

HIGHLY PROCESSED INGREDIENTS

(with a high concentration of additives, often listed on labels as E numbers)

HOW TO EAT WELL

GET YOUR NUTRIENTS

We should all take our nutrition seriously, so here are the benefits of vitamins and minerals that help to keep us healthy.

Vitamin A
Can improve vision / Helps your immune system
Butternut squash • carrots • spinach

Vitamin B12
Improved mood and energy levels / Maintains nerve cells
Nutritional yeast • yeast extract (we use Marmite) • some plant-based meat alternatives

Omega 3
Maintains a healthy cardiovascular system / Important for brain function
Walnuts • chia seeds • rapeseed oil

Vitamin D
Improves mental health / Can help prevent cancer / Good for bone health
Vitamin D-fortified mushrooms • fortified cereals • sunshine

Calcium
Good for brain function / Strengthens bones and teeth
Kale • tofu • almonds

Iron
Essential for good blood flow / Improves metabolism
Lentils • sweet potatoes • artichokes

Magnesium
Repairs and regenerates cells / Provides you with energy
Spinach • black beans • bananas

Zinc
Good for your immune system
Nuts • leafy green vegetables • oats

Fibre
Good for healthy gut bacteria / Makes it easier to manage weight
Berries • popcorn • wholegrain pasta

Iodine
Helps your thyroid gland to function properly
Fortified almond milk • seaweed • iodine supplements

GET YOUR PROTEIN

If you've started eating a plant-based diet, you're bound to wonder where you'll get your protein from. Here's a list of plant-based protein sources that can help.

Plant-based meat alternatives   Seitan, tofu and some shop-bought products

Legumes   Beans, peas and lentils

Grains   Brown rice, quinoa and bulgur wheat

Nuts   Almonds, brazils and peanuts

Seeds   Chia, sunflower and pumpkin

Vegetables   Leafy greens and potatoes

Spreads   Hummus, tahini and nut butter

Other   Spirulina, dark chocolate and plant-based protein powder

MEAT FEASTS

We've pulled together this neat little gallery of recipes to point you in the direction of some seriously delicious dishes for every situation, whether you're looking for something special to share with your partner, or something rich and spicy for an 'invite everyone you know' curry extravaganza.

DATE NIGHT

- Baked Tuna Puttanesca with Crispy Gnocchi (page 178)
- Creme Brûlée (page 230)
- Spicy Apricot Chickpeas and Lamb Tagine with Saffron Couscous (page 164)
- Chorizo Risotto (page 126)
- Lebanese-style Lamb Flatbreads with Minty Yoghurt (page 162)
- Date-night Scallops (page 174)
- Orzo Meatballs (page 84)
- Eton Mess (page 232)
- Spanakopita with Tomato and Pomegranate Za'atar Salad (page 208)

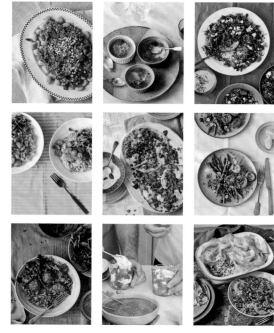

FAKEAWAY

- Crispy Shredded Beef with Egg-fried Rice (page 100)
- Crispy Korean-style Chicken Wings (page 46)
- Weeping Tiger Jay (page 124)
- Kung Pao Chicken (page 72)
- Pho King (page 114)
- Blackened Monk Chicken Noodles (page 54)
- Sausage Party Pizza (page 216)
- Pork Gyoza with Zippy Dippy (page 122)
- Duck Pancakes (page 70)

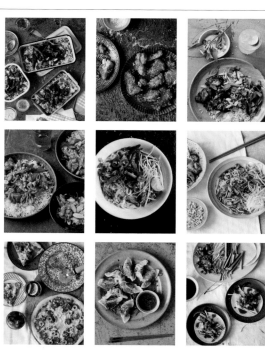

CURRY NIGHT

- **Meaty Bhuna and Aromatic Pilau Rice** (page 158)
- **Prawn Malai** (page 186)
- **Kare Raisu** (page 62)
- **Keema Paratha with Coconut Chutney** (page 86)
- **Kashmiri Lamb with Dum Aloo and Nigella Naan** (page 140)
- **Chicken Tikka Masala** (page 68)
- **Gaeng Phed Ped Yang with Coconut Rice** (page 58)

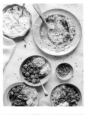
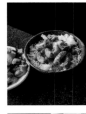
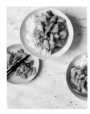
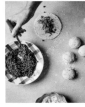
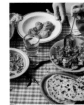
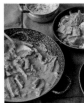
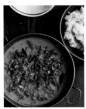

SARNIE SELECTION

- Lobster Roll (page 182)
- Pesto Chicken Sandwich (page 57)
- Fillet – WOAH – Fish (page 172)
- Philly Cheesesteak (page 78)
- BBQ Smash Burgers (page 98)
- KO Club Sandwich (page 74)
- Chippy's Hottest Dog (page 132)
- Shrimp Po'Boy (Fried Shrimp Sandwich) (page 192)
- Coronation Chicken Salad (page 60)

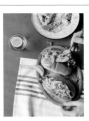
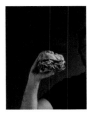
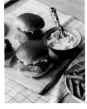
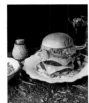
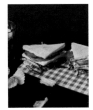
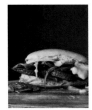
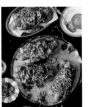
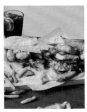
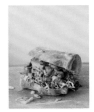

HOW TO MAKE MEAT

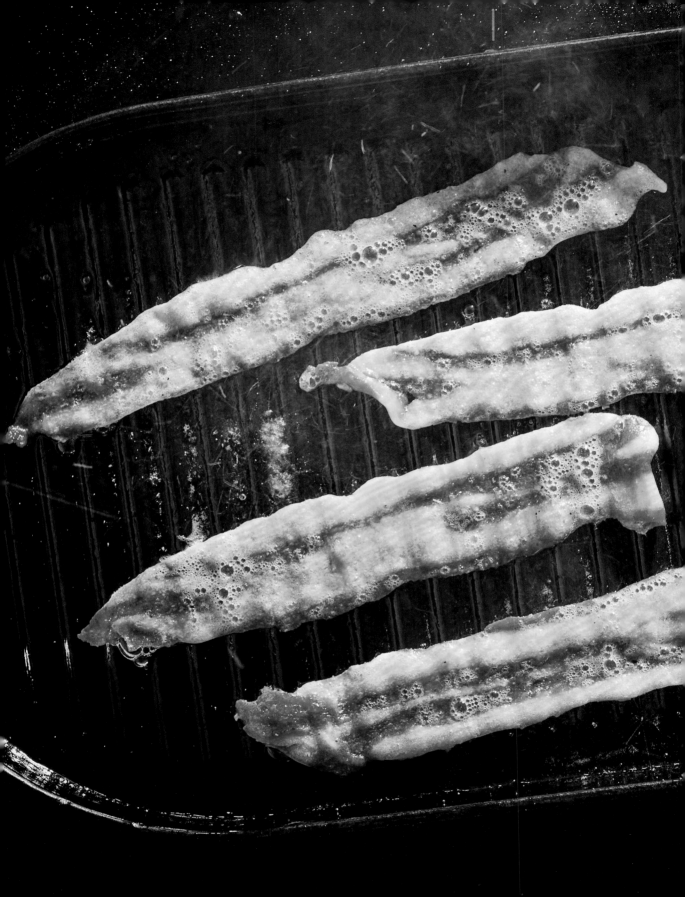

SAUSAGES

You've had a sausage but now's your chance to have a BOSHage. These purposely have a lovely simple flavour so, if you're feeling fancy, you can have a play with some seasonings and spices to make them your own.

MAKES 8 SAUSAGES

FOR THE WET INGREDIENTS
120g drained tinned chickpeas
200ml vegetable stock
80g aquafaba (chickpea tin water)
1 tbsp refined coconut oil
1 tbsp coconut aminos
1 tsp liquid smoke

FOR THE DRY INGREDIENTS
150g Vital wheat gluten flour
2 tbsp nooch (nutritional yeast)
1 tsp garlic powder
1 tbsp buckwheat flour
2 tbsp crispy fried onions
1 tsp beetroot powder

TO COOK THE SAUSAGES
vegetable oil

Powerful blender • Sandwich bags • Steaming pot and basket • Heavy-based frying pan

Blend the wet ingredients • Place all of the wet ingredients into a powerful blender and blend until smooth

Mix the dry ingredients together • Place all of the dry ingredients in a large mixing bowl and whisk until there are no lumps • Pour the wet mixture into the dry mixture and mix well until you have a rough dough • Remove the dough from the bowl and knead for 3 minutes on a work surface until strings start to form – it's important you don't overwork the dough or fold it like you would when making bread

Rest the dough • After 3 minutes, place the dough in a sandwich bag or wrap in cling film and leave to rest for 5 minutes

Shape the sausages • Once the dough has had time to rest, divide the mixture into 8 equal balls, each weighing about 70g • Roll each ball in your hands to make a rough sausage shape before wrapping them in cling film to shape the sausages • Tie each end of the cling film for each sausage to make a compact shape

Steam the sausages • Steam the sausages in a steaming basket for 35 minutes • After 35 minutes, cool the sausages a little before cooking or storing • If storing, place the sausages in the fridge

Cook the sausages • Once ready to cook the sausages, remove the cling film from each sausage • Place a heavy-based frying pan over a medium heat and add a drizzle of vegetable oil • Once warm, add the sausages • Slowly caramelise the sausages on all sides for 3–4 minutes, turning them constantly, until golden on the outsides and cooked through

NOTES
The beetroot powder makes the sausages bright red/pink when raw and brown once cooked.

The sausages will keep, well wrapped, for up to 5 days once cooked, or up to 3 months in the freezer.

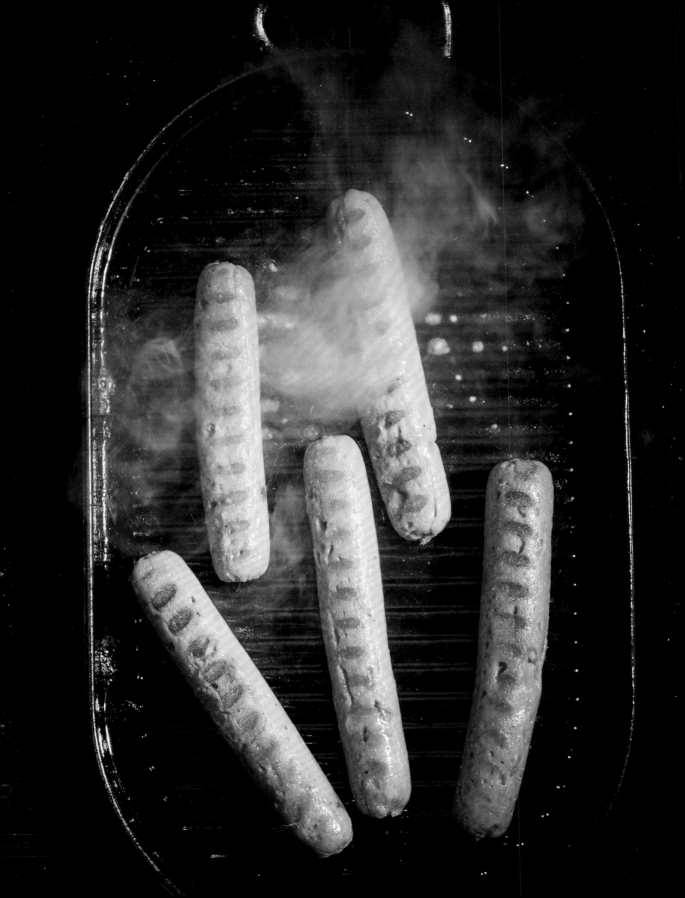

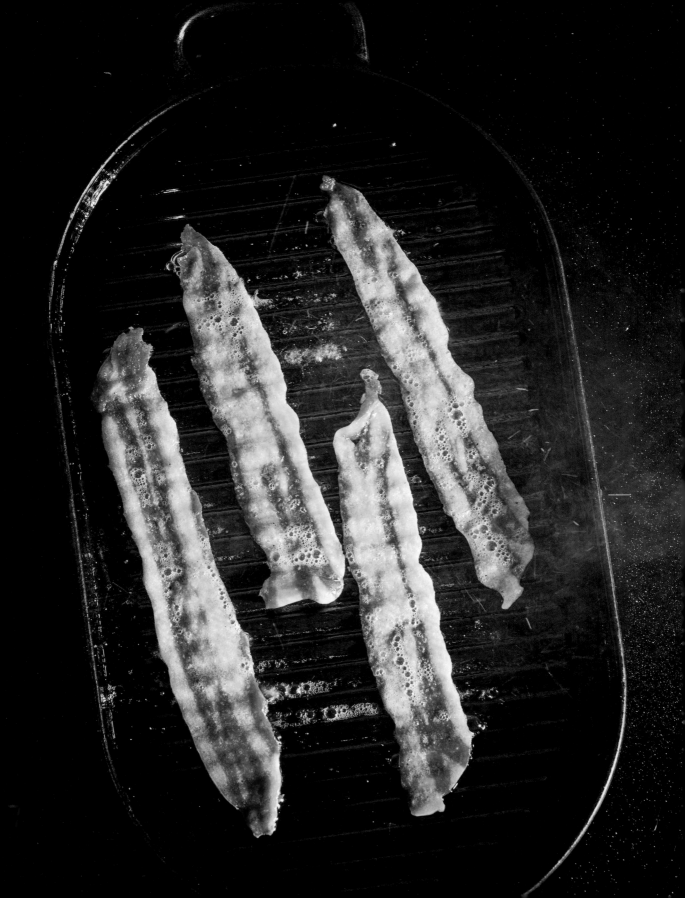

BACON

Good for a BLT, nice chopped into lardons, and perfect in a fry-up. This is the bacon recipe you've been searching for. It looks fantastic, it's got the texture you're after and it actually sizzles when it's frying. Make a batch of this – you'll be pleased you did!

MAKES 500G

FOR THE RED LAYER
160g drained chickpeas
120g aquafaba (chickpea
    tin water)
1 tsp garlic powder
2 tsp smoked paprika
1 tbsp mushroom powder
1 tbsp toasted sesame oil
10g nooch
    (nutritional yeast)
20g tomato purée
2 tsp liquid smoke
1 tsp cider vinegar
½ tsp agave syrup
20g white miso paste
2 tbsp beetroot powder
140g Vital wheat
    gluten flour

**FOR THE WHITE
LAYER**
120g aquafaba (chickpea
    tin water)
30g white miso paste
30g drained tinned
    chickpeas
140g Vital wheat
    gluten flour

TO COOK
refined coconut oil
sea salt and black pepper

Powerful food processor • Sandwich bags • Rolling pin • Large board • Long sharp knife • Large non-stick frying pan • Pastry brush

Make the red layer • Put all the ingredients, except the Vital wheat gluten flour, in a powerful food processor and blend until relatively smooth • Remove the mixture from the machine, add the wheat gluten flour and knead with your hands for 3 minutes • After kneading, divide the mixture in half and place each half into a sandwich bag • Leave to rest for 20 minutes while you make the white layer

Make the white layer • Clean out the bowl from making the red layer • Put all the ingredients, except the Vital wheat gluten flour, in a powerful food processor and blend until it all comes together • Remove the mixture from the machine, add the wheat gluten flour and knead with your hands for 3 minutes • After kneading, when the strands and fibres of the dough are visible as the gluten activates, divide the mixture in half and place each half into a sandwich bag • Leave to rest for 20 minutes

Roll the layers • Once both layers have been resting for 20 minutes, roll each of them into 2 x 5mm-thick rectangles – you should have 4 rectangles altogether

Assemble the bacon • On a large board, place one red rectangle down first • Place a white rectangle on top then repeat with another red rectangle and the final white rectangle on top • Season the whole thing with salt and black pepper

Freeze the bacon • Wrap the bacon in cling film and firm up in the freezer for at least 2 hours or even overnight

Shape the bacon • Once the bacon has firmed up slice it very thinly using a long sharp knife • Roll out each slice to make sure the bacon pieces are very thin

Cook the bacon • Place a large non-stick frying pan over a medium-low heat • Brush one side of the bacon slices with coconut oil • Once the pan is warm, add a few slices of the bacon, coconut-oil face down and cook for 5–6 minutes on one side • While one side is cooking, brush the top side with more coconut oil and season with sea salt • Once cooked, flip the bacon slices over and cook on the other side for 5–6 minutes until caramelised, brown and crispy – they will get more crispy once they are removed from the pan

Time to serve • Allow the bacon slices to rest for a few minutes before serving

NOTE
The block of bacon can be frozen for up to 3 months. It can also be sliced thinly and frozen in rashers. Freezing will affect the saltiness of the bacon, making it taste less seasoned, but this is added again during cooking. The bacon will keep in the fridge for 3 days (it may discolour after this).

CHICKEN

You've probably had plant-based chicken before, but we're willing to bet that it didn't have skin. This recipe includes an interesting technique to create crispy skin that we're sure you'll be impressed by. Make a great sandwich with it, use it as the meat in a roast dinner, or stir it into your curry to provide some super-satisfying meaty chunks. Whichever way you choose to use it, we hope you enjoy!

MAKES 4 CHICKEN BREASTS

FOR THE CHICKEN BREASTS
280g drained chickpeas (from a 400g tin)
100ml water
160g aquafaba (chickpea tin water)
2 tbsp plant-based chicken bouillon powder
1 tsp onion powder
1 tsp garlic powder
1 tbsp cider vinegar
1 tbsp white miso paste
240g Vital wheat gluten flour
sea salt and black pepper

FOR THE SOY-MILK CHICKEN SKIN
500ml unsweetened soy milk
plant-based chicken bouillon powder
sea salt and black pepper

Powerful food processor • Steamer set-up • Large saucepan • Chopsticks • Oven tray greased with oil • Frying pan • Baking tray

Make the chicken breasts • Put all of the chicken ingredients, except the Vital wheat gluten flour, in a powerful food processor and blend until the mixture becomes smooth • Pour the purée into a large mixing bowl and mix through the Vital wheat gluten flour until a rough dough forms • Remove the dough from the bowl and place onto a flat surface • Work the dough with your hands for 4 minutes until strings start to form • After 4 minutes, rest the dough for 5 minutes then cut it into 4 equal pieces • Shape each piece into a chicken breast shape and season all over with salt and pepper • Wrap each breast in cling film and steam for 45 minutes, taking care to not let the pan boil dry

Make the soy-milk skin • Bring the soy milk to the boil in a large saucepan over a medium heat, allowing a skin to form when it has raised up like one large thin and brittle bubble • Let the thin skin deflate back into the milk by turning off the heat and leave it to thicken for 3–4 minutes (it will thicken as it makes contact with the remaining milk) • Once it's visibly thickened, lift out the skin with chopsticks – try to avoid folding the sheet • Place the sheet on a pre-oiled baking tray and season with the chicken bouillon powder • Repeat the process once more

Cook the chicken • Once the chicken breasts have steamed, remove them from the steamer and allow them to cool before removing the cling film • Preheat oven to 180°C • Place the chicken breasts on the soy skin and cut around the breasts with a knife to make the skin the right size for each breast • Flip the skin over each breast and season with more chicken bouillon powder • Cook the breasts skin side down in a frying pan over a medium-high heat for 1–2 minutes to get a lovely caramelised colour • After browning, roast for 20–25 minutes in the oven on a baking tray (if you are using breasts straight from the fridge, allow them come up to room temperature 30 minutes before cooking) • Once cooked, rest on a chopping board for 5 minutes before slicing

NOTE
The chicken will keep in the fridge for up to 5 days or up to 3 months tightly wrapped in the freezer.

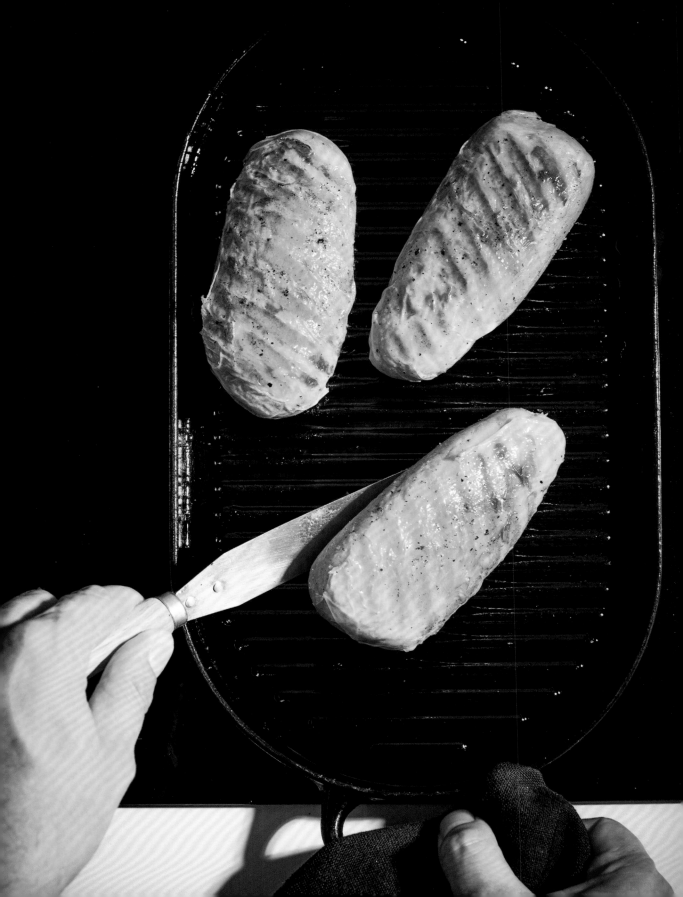

BEEF

In this section of the book, we were going to include base recipes for burgers and for steak but decided against it because this recipe does both really well. If you want a burger, shape the mixture into a patty, if you want a steak, shape the mixture into a steak. Simple. We think the texture of this beef is seriously impressive and we reckon you will too!

MAKES 6 BEEF STEAKS

**FOR THE
JACKFRUIT BROTH**
1 x 800g tin young green
    jackfruit in water
2 tbsp coconut oil
1 tbsp nooch
    (nutritional yeast)
1 tbsp treacle
1 tbsp yeast extract
    (we use Marmite)
3 tbsp cider vinegar
1 tbsp mushroom powder
1 tsp liquid smoke
250ml water
good pinch of sea salt

**FOR THE DRY
INGREDIENTS**
140g Vital wheat gluten flour
40g pea protein
2 tbsp tapioca starch
1 tbsp beetroot powder

FOR THE STEAKS
2 tbsp coconut oil
400ml boiling water
1 plant-based beef
    OXO cube
½ tsp yeast extract
    (we use Marmite)
olive oil, to serve
sea salt and black pepper

Potato masher • Colander or clean cloth • Large, deep frying pan with lid • Medium saucepan

Prepare the jackfruit • Drain the jackfruit and shred using your hands or two forks • Mash the pulled jackfruit with a potato masher until the fibres are fully separated • Place the mashed jackfruit into a colander or cloth and drain as much liquid from the mixture as possible – we leave it to sit for 10–15 minutes in the colander

Cook the jackfruit • Heat the coconut oil in a large, deep frying pan over a medium heat • Once melted, add the jackfruit and a good pinch of salt • Mix well and cook for 4 minutes • After 4 minutes, add the remaining broth ingredients and simmer very gently for 20 minutes • Turn off the heat and allow the broth to cool

Make the steaks • Drain the broth from the jackfruit, squeezing it out and reserving all of the liquid in a saucepan • In a large bowl, mix together the dry ingredients • Add the jackfruit mixture and mix well then add a dash of the broth, bit-by-bit, until you have a nice dough • Remove the dough from the bowl and place onto a flat surface • Knead the dough for 3–4 minutes until strings start to form • Divide the dough into 6 equal pieces and shape into a steak shape • Wrap each steak in cling film and leave in the fridge for at least 1 hour

Cook the steaks • Unwrap the steaks and season each with salt and pepper • Place a large, deep frying pan over a medium-high heat and add the coconut oil • Once hot, sear the steaks for 3–4 minutes on each side until golden and you get a nice crispy caramelisation • In a small bowl, mix 400ml of boiling water with the stock cube and yeast extract • Pour in any remaining cooking broth and mix again • Pour the liquid over the steaks and leave to simmer for 20 minutes with the lid on, flipping the steaks occasionally

Leave to rest • After 20 minutes, leave the steaks to rest for a few minutes on a board before slicing

Time to serve • Serve the steaks with the cooking juices and a good glug of olive oil

NOTE
The beef will keep for up to 3 days wrapped in the fridge, or individually wrapped in the freezer for up to 3 months.

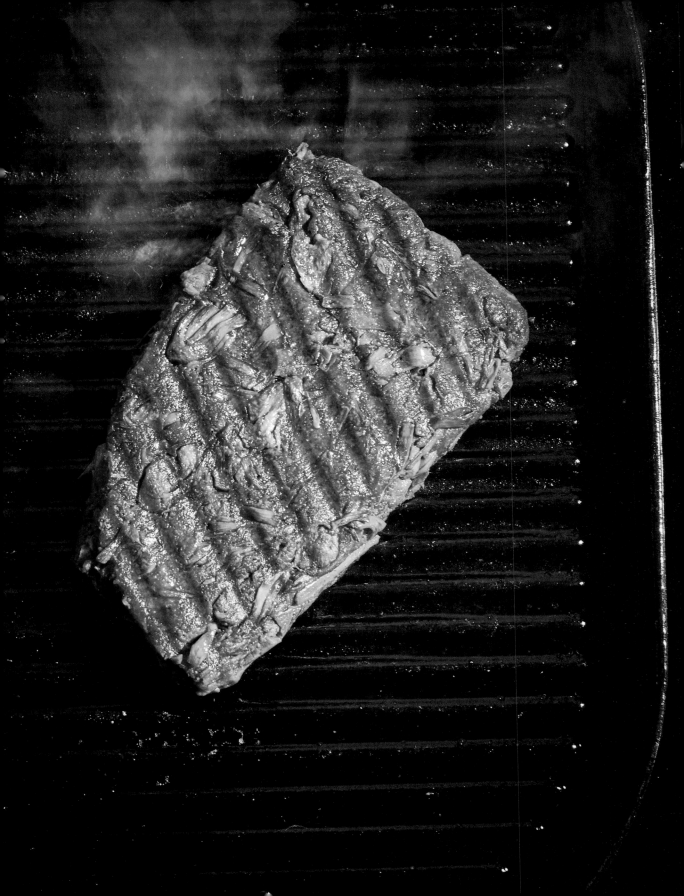

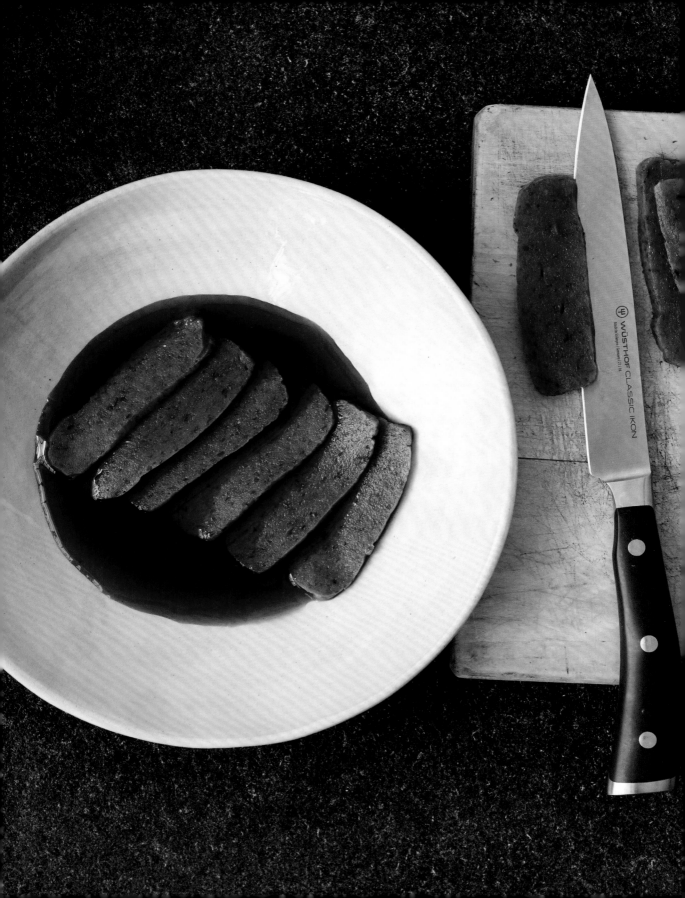

FISH (TUNA)

Delicate, surprising, interesting... We really like this recipe because it's so different from anything else in this book; it's kinda like a properly firm savoury jelly that slices really nicely. It's not like tuna from a tin, more like a tuna or swordfish steak. Serve it in a salad, with rice, or in sushi, and we're sure your guests will be impressed!

MAKES 6 BLOCKS FOR SUSHI

FOR THE FIRST GEL
2 tsp konjac gum/flour
230ml water
⅛ tsp red food colouring
1 tsp seaweed flakes
pinch of salt
1 tbsp Nish fish sauce

FOR THE ALKALINE SOLUTION
¼ tsp bicarbonate of soda
100ml water

FOR THE SECOND GEL
1 tsp agar agar powder
3 tbsp tapioca starch
100ml water

FOR THE MARINADE
1 tbsp mirin
3 tbsp light soy sauce
juice of ½ lemon

Whisk • Medium saucepan • Silicone mat with 6 deep silicone moulds • Large, deep frying pan

Make the first gel • Place the konjac gum in a large mixing bowl • Slowly and carefully pour in the water, whisking constantly to avoid any lumps • Once the mixture has come together, whisk in the remaining 'first gel' ingredients • Simmer the mixture in a saucepan for about 6 minutes to dissolve the konjac, whisking constantly, then leave to cool and transfer to the fridge

Add the alkaline solution • In a small bowl, whisk together the bicarbonate of soda and water • Pour the mixture into the chilled 'first gel' solution and whisk well to incorporate • Place in the fridge until it cools, then pour the mixture into a medium saucepan

Add the second gel • Add the agar agar, tapioca starch and water to the saucepan with the other ingredients • Bring to the boil, then reduce the temperature and simmer for 6 minutes to activate the agar agar • Turn off the heat and allow to cool slightly before pouring into silicone moulds

Cook the mixture • Place the silicone mat of moulds filled with the tuna solution in a large, deep frying pan and pour in enough boiling water so that the level of the water is nearly reaching the top of the moulds (similar to a bain-marie) • Gently simmer over a low heat for 20 minutes • After 20 minutes, transfer to the fridge and refrigerate for at least 2 hours

Time to serve • Mix all of the marinade ingredients together and serve with the tuna – the tuna can sit within the marinade or the marinade can be poured on top before serving • Thinly slice the tuna and serve in your favourite dishes

NOTE
The 'tuna' in this recipe can be used in a variety of different ways. Some examples include; cut up and used in marinated tartare with avocado, on/ within sushi rolls or sliced and used as sashimi.

CHEDDAR

It grates, it slices, it melts and it's super-cheesy. This is the homemade plant-based cheese recipe you've been looking for. If you want to have a play around by popping in some herbs and spices, feel free! Getting creative in the kitchen is fun and will help you improve as a cook.

MAKES 400G

25g raw unsalted cashews
400g full-fat coconut milk
3 tbsp nooch
    (nutritional yeast)
1 tsp sea salt
1 tbsp cider vinegar
1 tbsp white miso paste
2 tsp Dijon mustard
⅛ tsp turmeric
2½ tsp agar agar powder
    or kappa carrageenan
100ml water

Medium saucepan • Kettle boiled • Powerful blender • Small saucepan • Container or mould for the cheese

Soak the cashews • Place the cashews in a medium saucepan over a medium heat and cover with boiling water • Simmer for 20 minutes • After 20 minutes, drain the cashews

Blend the ingredients • Put the drained cashews, coconut milk, nooch, salt, cider vinegar, white miso, Dijon mustard and turmeric in a powerful blender • Pulse quickly and blend together until smooth

Cook the agar agar • Place the agar agar in a small saucepan over a medium heat and add the 100ml water • Simmer for 6 minutes to activate, topping up with a little more water if needed

Form the cheese • Put the agar agar water with the rest of the ingredients in the blender and blend • Once smooth, pour the mixture into your container or mould, banging it on the worktop to remove the bubbles that will have formed

Set the cheese • Allow the cheese to cool at room temperature for 20 minutes • After 20 minutes, wrap the cheese in cling film and set in the fridge until needed

NOTE
The cheddar will keep in the fridge for up to 5 days, or in the freezer, well wrapped, for up to 3 months.

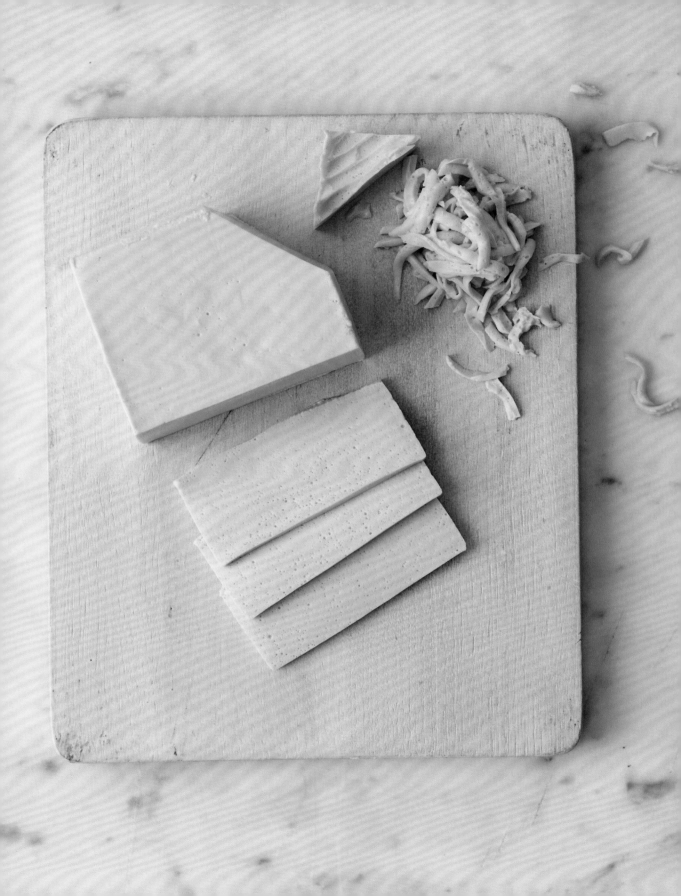

MILK

The lovely creamy texture and lush subtle flavour of this milk makes it perfect to splash on your cereal before you head off to work. Enjoy!

**MAKES 1 LITRE
OAT MILK**

6 medjool dates
200g rolled oats
1.5 litres filtered water
pinch of sea salt

Powerful blender • Cheesecloth • Funnel • 1-litre bottle, jug or airtight container

Prepare the milk • Pit the dates and roughly cut into small pieces • Add the oats, dates, water and salt to a powerful blender and blend until smooth

Strain the milk • Pour the liquid into a jug, bottle or container through a cheesecloth to catch all the sediment and twist any remaining liquid out of the pulp into the container • If the milk is too thick, you can mix through a dash of water until it reaches the consistency you like best

Store the milk • Cover the container, store in the fridge and consume within 5 days • Make sure you shake the container or stir the milk every time you want to use the milk

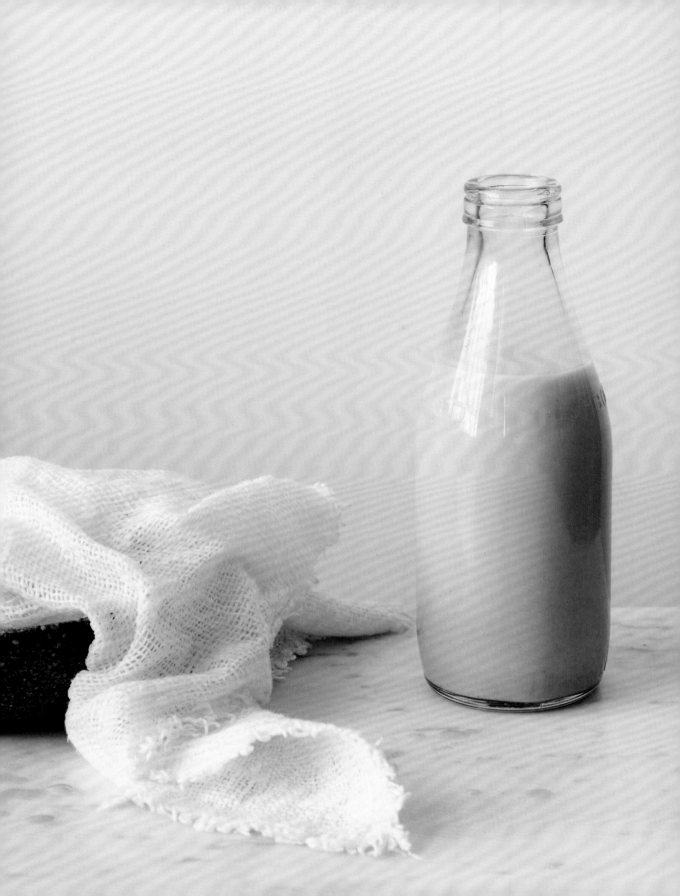

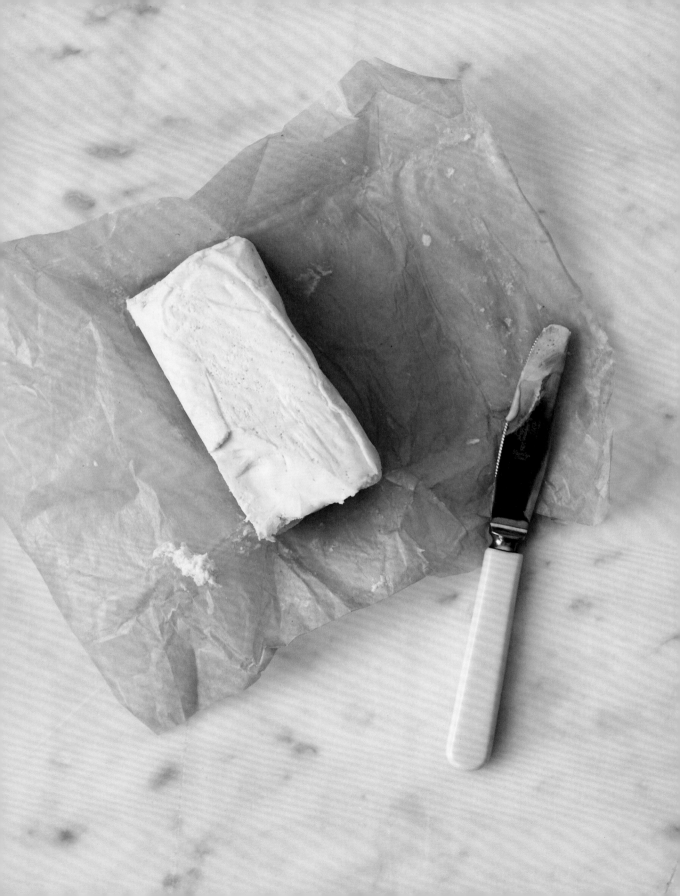

BUTTER

Spread it on your toast, whack a knob in your jacket tatties or lump a little into your curry to give it a delicious silky edge. This butter has a lovely subtle flavour, glorious viscous mouthfeel and robust density; a fantastic homemade replacement to store-bought varieties.

MAKES 400G

130g unsweetened soy milk, at room temperature
1 tsp cider vinegar
150g refined coconut oil
50g cold-pressed rapeseed oil
1 tsp nooch (nutritional yeast)
⅛–½ tsp turmeric (the more you add, the more yellow the butter will be)
¼ tsp sea salt
5g soy lecithin powder (optional, see Note)

Powerful blender • Baking paper • 2 butter block-sized containers

Make a buttermilk • Pour the room-temperature soy milk and cider vinegar into a large mixing bowl and allow to curdle for 5–10 minutes

Blend the ingredients to make the butter • Put the refined coconut oil and rapeseed oil in a powerful blender and blend until the liquids come together • Add the curdled milk and all of the remaining ingredients and blend until completely emulsified – no more than 1 minute

Set the butter • Immediately pour the mixture into 2 butter block-sized containers to set

Time to serve • After about an hour, once the butter has set, wrap in baking paper to store or serve in a butter dish • If storing, store in the fridge for up to a month, well wrapped

NOTE
The soy lecithin powder in this recipe is to fully set the butter and ensure it doesn't split when it melts. If you can't get any, you can make this recipe without the ingredient, it will still set in the fridge but will be a little softer and may separate when fully melted.

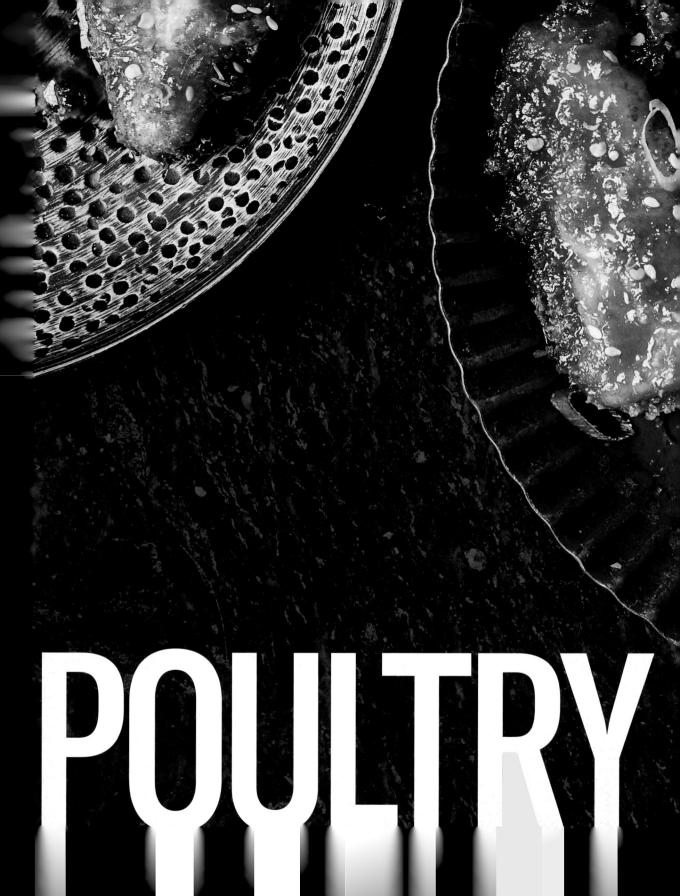

POULTRY

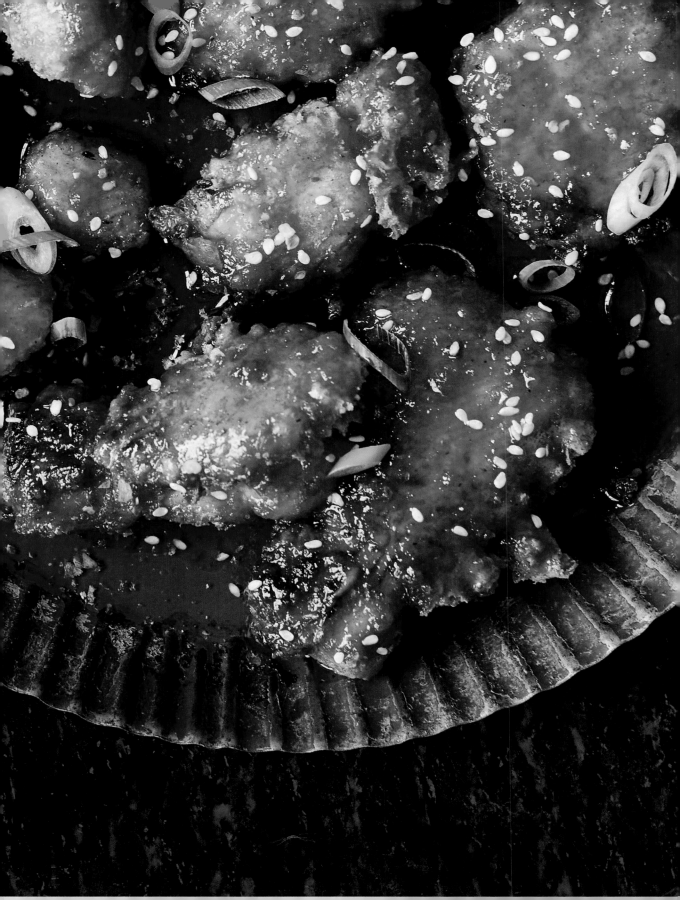

CRISPY KOREAN-STYLE CHICKEN WINGS

These wings are SO crispy and delicious! Seriously, we love them. You can eat them as they come or you could push the boat out and serve them in a sandwich with a little plant-based mayo, kimchi and lettuce with a side of fries. They'd also go well with a side of rice and a little salad. Whichever way you choose, we're pretty sure you'll love them as much as we do.

SERVES 4–6 AS A SIDE

FOR THE STICKY MARINADE
4 garlic cloves
2.5cm piece of fresh ginger
150g gochujang
120ml toasted sesame oil
2 tbsp rice vinegar
2 tbsp light soy sauce
4 tbsp light brown sugar
¼ tsp ground white pepper

FOR THE CHICKEN
2 x 280g blocks
   extra-firm tofu
6 tbsp cornflour
½ tsp sea salt
¼ tsp ground white pepper
vegetable oil, for
   shallow frying

FOR THE GARNISH
1 fresh chilli or a pinch of
   dried chilli flakes
1 spring onion
a few toasted sesame
   seeds, for sprinkling

Fine grater or microplane • Blender (optional) • Frying pan • Saucepan • Line a plate or large bowl with kitchen paper

Make the marinade • Peel the garlic and ginger and grate with a fine grater or microplane • Combine with the rest of the ingredients and either blitz in a blender or combine in a bowl and stir into a nice smooth paste

Prepare the chicken • Press the tofu to remove excess liquid • Tear the tofu into rough chunks about 3 x 2cm • Add the tofu to a mixing bowl along with half the marinade and fold to coat • Sprinkle the cornflour, salt and pepper into the bowl and fold to coat and combine, making sure the tofu is really well covered

Cook the chicken • Pour 1cm of oil into a frying pan and heat over a medium-high heat until the oil bubbles around the end of a wooden spoon that's held in the oil • Carefully lower the tofu chunks into the hot oil and cook for 2–3 minutes until golden and crispy, turning them regularly to ensure a really even cook • Remove carefully and drain on a plate lined with kitchen paper

Finish the dish • Put the remaining marinade into a saucepan, bring to a simmer and cook until thick and shiny • Add the cooked tofu to the sauce and quickly fold it through to ensure a good coverage • Spoon the tofu into a serving bowl • Trim and thinly slice the spring onion for the garnish and finely chop the chilli (if using fresh chilli) • Garnish the tofu with the chilli or chilli flakes, spring onion and toasted sesame seeds and serve immediately with some cold beers!

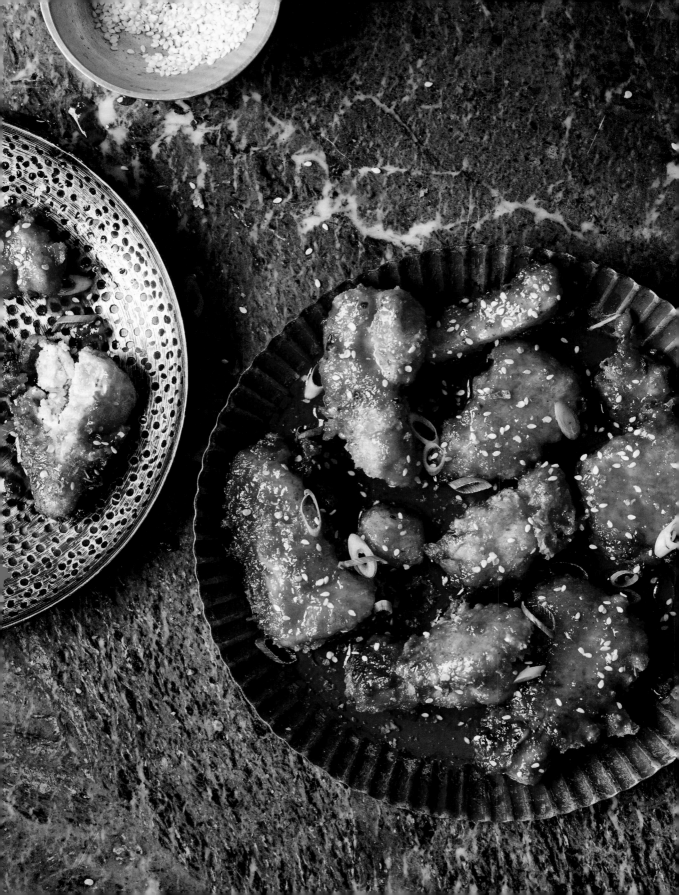

CREAMY RED PEPPER PENNE

A creamy cashew sauce blended with nooch (nutritional yeast) and lemon juice to give it that delicious cheesy flavour, mixed through pasta layered with sun-dried tomatoes, plant-based chicken pieces and spinach – absolute heaven. We've called this Creamy Red Pepper Penne, but to be honest it works with any pasta shape you have in the cupboard. In fact, the sauce works really well with wheat-free pasta like lentil or rice pasta too. If you like pasta as much as we do (which is a lot) we urge you to make a mental note of this recipe because we think there's a high chance that you'll come back to it time and time again!

SERVES 4

FOR THE SAUCE
150g raw unsalted cashews
200ml unsweetened
    almond milk
30g nooch
    (nutritional yeast)
1 tbsp Dijon mustard
1 lemon
sea salt

FOR THE PASTA
1 onion
2 garlic cloves
2 red peppers
good drizzle of olive oil
1 small jar of sun-dried
    tomatoes
1 tsp paprika
1 tsp dried mixed herbs
1 x 160g pack plant-based
    chicken pieces
250g penne pasta
220g baby spinach
sea salt

TO SERVE
handful of cherry tomatoes
nooch (nutritional yeast),
    to taste
flat-leaf parsley
black pepper

Kettle boiled • Large high-sided frying pan • Powerful blender • Large saucepan

Soak the cashews • Place the cashews in a heatproof bowl and cover with boiling water • Leave to one side for at least 1 hour until needed

Make the pasta base • Peel and dice the onion and garlic • Halve and core the peppers and cut into small cubes • Place a large high-sided frying pan over a medium heat and add the olive oil (we use the oil from the sun-dried tomato jar) • Drain and chop the sun-dried tomatoes • Once the oil's warm, add the diced onion, garlic and a pinch of salt • Mix well and cook for 5–10 minutes, or until the onion begins to soften • Add the red peppers and sun-dried tomatoes, mix well and cook for another 10 minutes • Add the paprika, dried herbs and plant-based chicken pieces into the pan and cook for as long as it states on the packet (about 5 minutes)

Make the sauce • Drain the cashews and place them into a powerful blender along with the almond milk, nooch, mustard and a pinch of salt • Halve the lemon and squeeze in the juice, catching any pips with your free hand • Blend until smooth, adding a dash more almond milk if needed

Cook the pasta • Bring a large saucepan of salted water to the boil • Once boiling, add the pasta and cook for 1 minute less than stated on the pack • Once cooked, drain the pasta (saving some of the pasta water to mix through later) and return to the pan

Finish the pasta • Roughly chop the spinach, add to the pasta base and cook until it wilts • Pour the sauce into the pan with the pasta and cook for a few minutes until heated through • Add a dash of pasta water to make the sauce really creamy and cook for a few more minutes until everything is piping hot

Time to serve • Quarter the tomatoes and scatter them on top of the pasta, along with a good sprinkle of nooch, a pinch of pepper and chop some parsley for sprinkling at the end

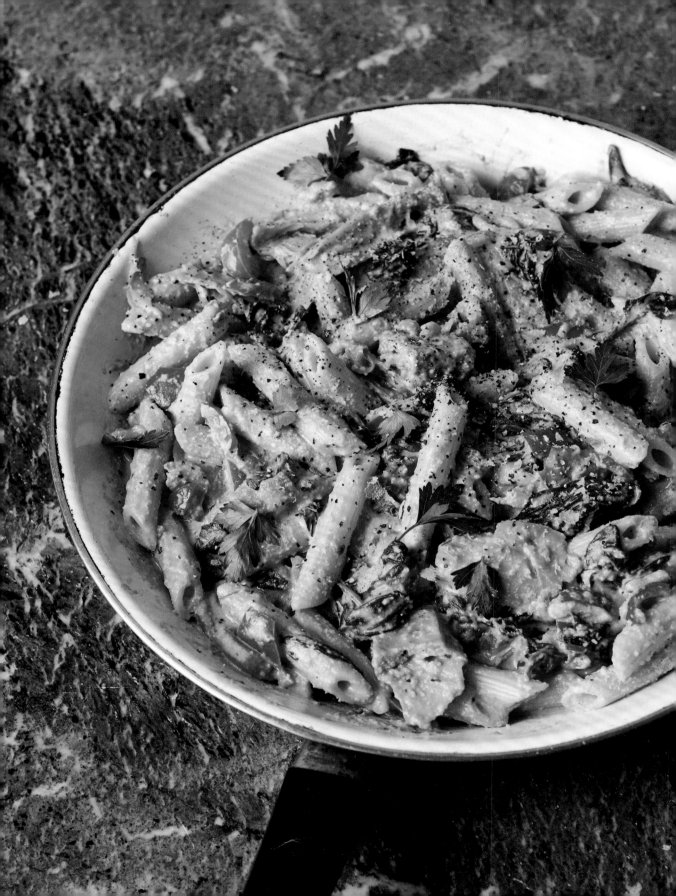

CHEESY CHICKEN ENCHILADAS AND MEXICAN-STYLE CORN SALAD

We're absolutely convinced that if you made a huge vat of this enchilada sauce, bottled it and sold it at your local food market, you'd sell out pretty quickly because it's outrageously tasty.

If you've never tried enchiladas before, we strongly recommend you mark this page with a sticky note immediately! The mixture of plant-based cheeses creates the perfect stringy enchiladas in this dish and complements the spicy filling. It's all served with a corn, lime and red onion salad that will blow your mind.

SERVES 4

FOR THE ROASTED INGREDIENTS
1 x 280g tin jackfruit in water
2 red, or red and
    yellow, peppers
½ aubergine
1 x pack plant-based
    chicken pieces
    (about 160g)
3 tbsp olive oil
2 tsp salt

FOR THE ENCHILADA SAUCE
250g tomatoes on the vine
4 tbsp olive oil
2 tbsp red wine vinegar
1 tsp sea salt
5 dried chipotle chillies
1 large onion
4 garlic cloves
2 tbsp maple syrup
1 tbsp ground cumin
2 tsp dried oregano
1 tsp smoked paprika
1 tsp ground cinnamon
150ml dry sherry
150ml water
95g smoked chipotle sauce

FOR THE ENCHILADA FILLING
1 x 400g tin black beans
1 lemon
bunch of oregano leaves
20g fresh parsley leaves
1 tbsp olive oil
200g plant-based
    grated cheddar
200g plant-based
    grated mozzarella
8 large corn tortillas
sea salt

Preheat oven to 200°C • 2 roasting trays • Kettle boiled • Large frying pan • Blender

Prepare the roasting ingredients • Wash, drain and pat-dry the jackfruit • Put the jackfruit in a roasting tray and crush the chunks between your fingers to split the fibres • Remove any seeds (they look a little like cannellini beans) • Halve, core and thinly slice the peppers • Trim and cut the aubergine into 1cm cubes • Add the peppers, aubergine and plant-based chicken pieces to the roasting tray, drizzle with the olive oil, sprinkle with the salt, stir to coat, then place in the oven and roast for 30 minutes, stirring halfway through

Prepare the sauce • Put the tomatoes, 2 tablespoons of the olive oil, the vinegar and salt in a second roasting tray and stir to coat • Roast in the oven for 30 minutes • Put the chipotle chillies in a jug and cover with boiling water to hydrate • Peel and dice the onion and garlic • Warm the remaining olive oil in a large frying pan over a low-medium heat, add the onion and garlic and sweat for 12–15 minutes until soft • Add the maple syrup, ground cumin, dried oregano, smoked paprika and ground cinnamon to the pan and cook for a couple of minutes • Add the soaked and drained chillies, sherry, water and chipotle sauce to the pan, reduce the heat to a gentle simmer and cook for 20–25 minutes • Add the roasted tomatoes to the pan, fold to combine, take off the heat and leave to cool to room temperature • Transfer the cooled contents of the pan to a blender and blitz into a smooth sauce

Prepare the filling • Drain the black beans and tip them into a bowl • Halve the lemon • Pick the oregano and parsley leaves and roughly chop • Squeeze the lemon juice over the beans (catching any pips in your free hand), add the olive oil, cheese, herbs and stir to combine • Taste and season to perfection with salt

Finish the filling • Transfer the roasted ingredients and a third of the sauce to the black beans and fold to combine

Build the enchiladas • Tightly roll an eighth of the filling in a tortilla and lay it in the roasting tray • Repeat until all the enchiladas are filled and neatly nestled in the tray • Drizzle the remaining sauce down the middle of the enchiladas, put the tray in the oven and roast for 20 minutes

FOR THE
CORN SALAD
1 x 570g tin sweetcorn
1 tbsp olive oil
2 tsp sea salt
1 red onion
2 green peppers
6 spring onions
4 large green chillies
30g coriander leaves
100g lettuce
2 limes
1 tbsp plant-based
    mayonnaise
1 tsp cayenne pepper

TO SERVE
handful of chives
handful of coriander
    leaves

Make the salad • Rinse and drain the sweetcorn and add to a bowl with the olive oil and 1 teaspoon of the salt • Peel and finely dice the onion • Halve, core and dice the peppers • Trim and thinly slice the spring onions • Halve, deseed and finely dice the chillies • Pick and thinly slice the coriander leaves • Shred the lettuce • Halve the limes and squeeze the juice over the corn • Add all the ingredients to the bowl and fold to coat • Add the mayo, cayenne and remaining salt and fold to combine

Time to serve • Chop the chives for the garnish and pick the coriander leaves • Transfer 2 enchiladas to each plate, dress with the corn salad, garnish with coriander and chopped chives and serve immediately

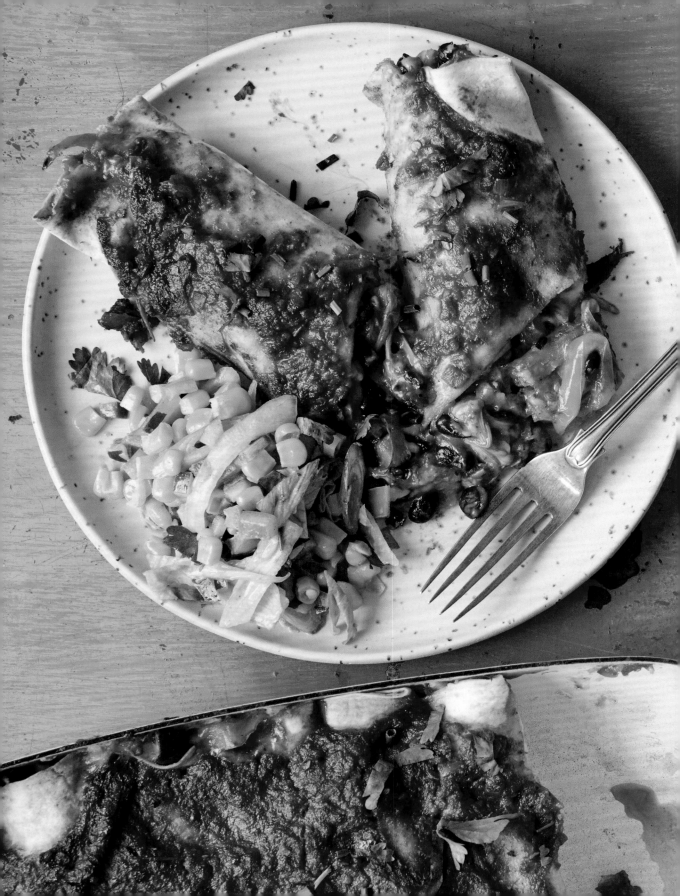

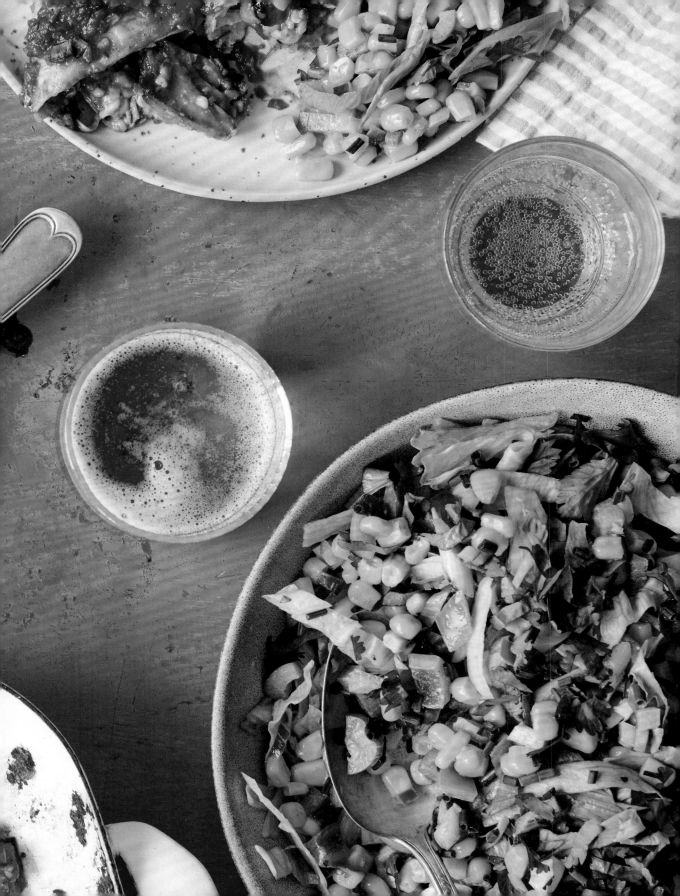

BLACKENED MONK CHICKEN NOODLES

During lockdown we lived with our mate Darren in an area of London called Clapham. During this time, to cheer us up, we ordered a fair few takeaways. One of the takeaways we ordered the most was Blackened Monk Noodles from a restaurant called Banana Tree: thick glass noodles and red onion coated in a rich sauce made from black beans, miso and tamari, served with a simple carrot and daikon pickle and a sprinkle of salted peanuts for an extra crunch. This is our take on a dish that put smiles on our faces numerous times during lockdown – we hope it puts a smile on your face too!

SERVES 2

FOR THE PICKLE
1 large carrot
1 daikon (about 400g)
1 tbsp table salt
375ml boiling water
5 tbsp caster sugar
4 tbsp distilled white vinegar

FOR THE SAUCE
150g black bean sauce
2 tsp brown rice miso paste
1½ tbsp tamari
1 tbsp rice vinegar
1 tbsp toasted sesame oil
sea salt

FOR THE NOODLES
1 small head of broccoli
drizzle of olive oil
100g folded rice noodles
1 red onion
drizzle of toasted sesame oil
1 x pack plant-based
    chicken pieces
    (about 160g)
100g beansprouts
sea salt

TO SERVE (ALL OPTIONAL)
1 or 2 limes
handful of coriander leaves
50g salted peanuts
1 red chilli
handful of plant-based
    prawn crackers
sprinkle of sesame seeds

Sterilised jam jar (or a large bowl) • Baking tray • Small saucepan • Large saucepan

Make the pickle • Peel and thinly slice the carrot and daikon, or cut them into matchsticks, and place in a bowl • Add the salt, mix well and leave for 20 minutes • After 20 minutes, rinse the vegetables well to remove the salt and spoon into a sterilised jam jar (or a large bowl) • Mix the boiling water with the sugar and vinegar until all of the sugar has dissolved • Pour the pickling liquid into the jar with the vegetables • Cover and leave to pickle (for the best results, leave for 2–3 days; for a quick pickle, leave for at least 2 hours)

Make the sauce • In a small mixing bowl, mix together the black bean sauce, brown rice miso paste, tamari, rice vinegar, toasted sesame oil and a pinch of salt until smooth

Cook the broccoli • Preheat oven to 180°C • Cut the broccoli into small florets and place on a baking tray • Drizzle with olive oil and season with a pinch of salt • Mix well and roast for 15–20 minutes until cooked through

Cook the noodles • Cook the noodles in a small saucepan according to the instructions on the packet • Once cooked, drain and rinse under cold running water to prevent the noodles from sticking together

Finish the sauce • Peel and roughly slice the red onion • Place a large saucepan over a medium heat and add the toasted sesame oil • Once warm, add the onion and a pinch of salt • Mix well and cook for 5 minutes until the onion starts to soften • Stir through the plant-based chicken pieces and cook for another 3 minutes, or until the plant-based chicken pieces have browned on the outside • Mix through the beansprouts and cook for another 5 minutes before pouring in the sauce and leaving to simmer for a few minutes

Finish the noodles • Add the roasted broccoli florets and cooked noodles to the saucepan • Mix well and cook for a further 5 minutes until everything is piping hot and coated in sauce

Time to serve • Slice the lime(s) into wedges • Chop the coriander and peanuts, slice the red chilli • Spoon the noodles onto serving plates • Drain the pickle and serve on the side of the noodles, along with a lime wedge, a handful of chopped peanuts and some prawn crackers • Top the two servings with sliced red chilli, chopped coriander, peanuts and a sprinkle of sesame seeds

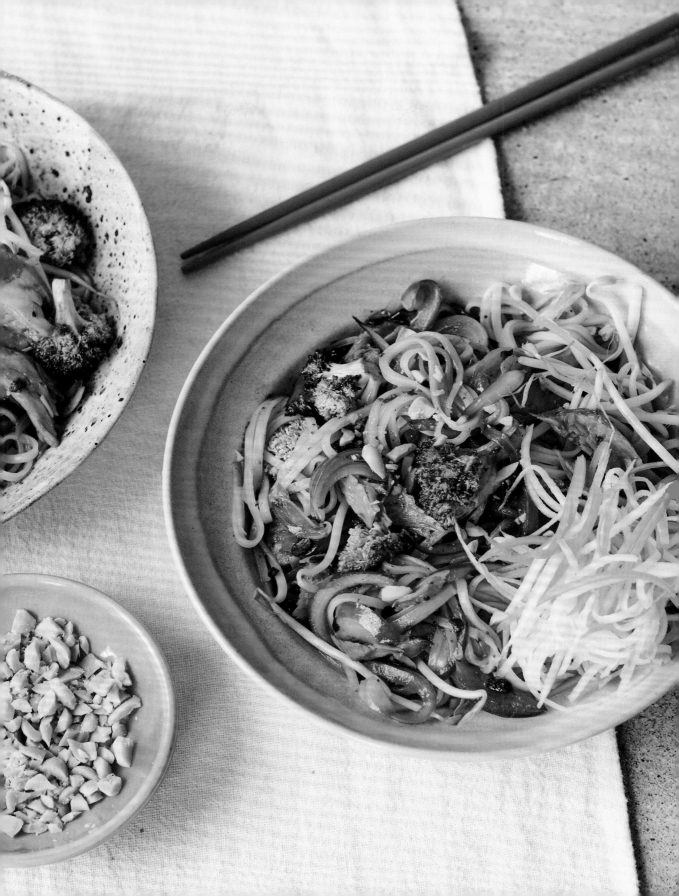

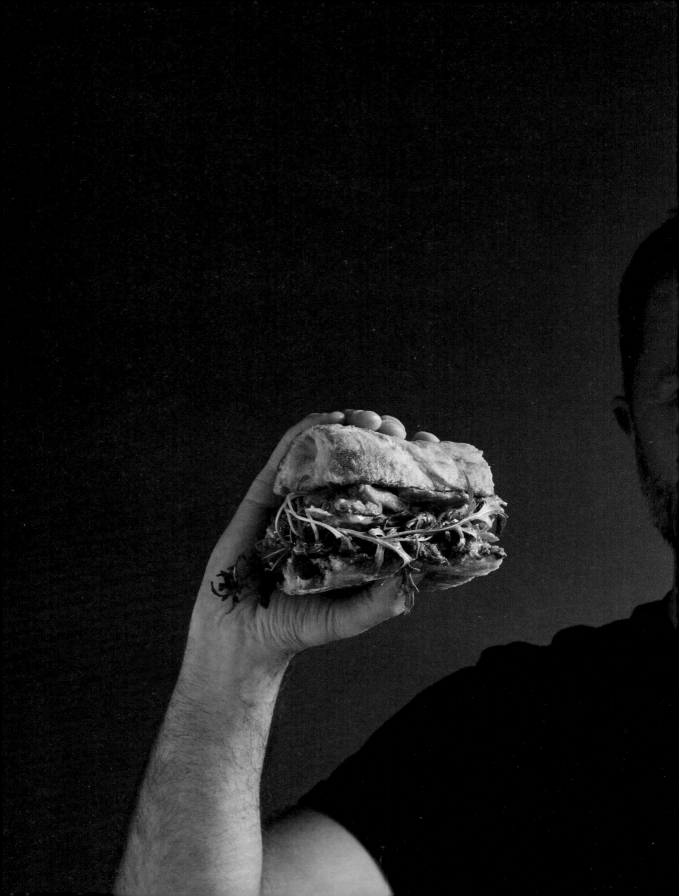

PESTO CHICKEN SANDWICH

If you like pesto you're gonna need to make these sandwiches. They're simple, quick and downright delicious. Seriously, this is one of those recipes that just paints a smile on your face. Serve on a sunny afternoon with a cold drink and you'll be as happy as Larry (we're not sure who Larry is but we're glad he's happy).

SERVES 4

FOR THE PESTO
50g pine nuts
50g fresh basil
1 garlic clove
1 tbsp nooch
   (nutritional yeast)
50g plant-based mozzarella
200ml extra-virgin olive oil
sea salt

FOR THE SANDWICH
2 large ciabatta loaves
drizzle of olive oil
480g plant-based
   chicken pieces
100g plant-based
   mayonnaise
1 tbsp Dijon mustard
½ lemon

TO SERVE
2 small sun-dried tomatoes
100g rocket
crisps

Preheat oven to 180°C • Small baking sheet • Food processor • Large frying pan

Make the pesto • Spread the pine nuts out on a small baking sheet and toast in the oven for 5 minutes • Pick the basil leaves off the stalks and put the leaves in a food processor along with the toasted pine nuts and blitz to a paste • Peel and grate the garlic clove into the processor, add the nooch and mozzarella and pulse again • Remove the blade from the processor and stir in enough of the oil to bind • Taste and season to perfection with salt

Prepare the ciabatta • Toast the ciabatta in the oven for 8–12 minutes until lightly golden and crisp • Cut both loaves into two sandwiches • Drizzle with a good glug of olive oil and return to the oven until golden and crispy on both sides then set to one side

Prepare the chicken • Heat a drizzle of olive oil in a large frying pan over a medium-high heat, add the plant-based chicken pieces and sauté for a couple of minutes (or according to the packet instructions) to cook through and colour them slightly • Transfer to a mixing bowl along with the mayo, 160g of the pesto, the Dijon mustard and a good squeeze of lemon juice, catching any pips in your free hand • Fold everything together, taste and season to perfection if necessary

Time to serve • Thinly slice the sun-dried tomatoes • Build the sandwiches with the tomatoes, rocket and pesto chicken and serve immediately with crisps and a cold beer

NOTE
Keep any leftover pesto in the fridge in an airtight container and use it in other recipes.

GAENG PHED PED YANG WITH COCONUT RICE

BIG flavours and BIG textures combine to form a BIG meal that will delight all who make it. Thai cuisine is right up there as one of the tastiest, and we think this recipe proves it. The coconut rice is soft and creamy, making the perfect base for the spiced, aromatic curry sauce made from fresh ginger, red Thai curry paste and coconut milk. The mock duck is coated in the sauce and melts in your mouth with the most moreish texture.

SERVES 4

FOR THE COCONUT RICE
300g Thai sticky rice
350ml boiling water
40g desiccated coconut
160ml coconut cream
½ tsp sea salt
1 tsp caster sugar

FOR THE CURRY SAUCE
1 onion
25g fresh ginger
3 garlic cloves
drizzle of toasted sesame oil
3 tbsp red Thai curry paste
2 tbsp apple purée
1 x 400g tin coconut milk
100ml water
200g tinned chopped
	tomatoes
2 tsp plant-based
	Thai fish sauce
1 tsp brown sugar
2 tsp light soy sauce
5 fresh makrut lime leaves
5g Thai basil leaves

FOR THE DUCK
drizzle of toasted sesame oil
560g plant-based shredded
	mock duck
½ tsp sea salt
2 tsp Chinese five-spice
1 orange

TO SERVE
3 spring onions
2 red chillies
Thai basil leaves

Powerful blender • 2 large frying pans • Large saucepan and lid • Tongs

Prepare the rice • Soak the rice in cold water while you make the sauce

Make the curry sauce • Peel and roughly chop the onion, ginger and garlic • Place in a powerful blender with a pinch of salt and blend until they break down and come together to form a paste • Heat the toasted sesame oil in a large frying pan over a medium heat • Once hot, add the onion, ginger and garlic mixture, curry paste and apple purée • Mix well and cook for a couple of minutes then add the coconut milk, water, the tinned tomatoes, fish sauce, sugar, soy sauce, lime leaves and Thai basil leaves • Mix well and cook for 30 minutes

Cook the duck • Heat the toasted sesame oil in a second large frying pan over a medium heat • Once hot, add the duck with the salt and Chinese five-spice • Mix well and cook for 4–8 minutes until the duck has browned, turning it every so often with tongs • Once the duck has turned brown, halve the orange, squeeze in the juice and mix through • Shred the duck into smaller chunks with two forks and set aside while you cook the rice

Cook the rice • Drain the rice from the water it is soaking in • Place a large saucepan over a medium heat and add the 350ml of boiling water • Add the drained rice, desiccated coconut, coconut cream, salt and sugar and mix well • Bring to the boil then place the lid on top, reduce the heat to low and cook for 10 minutes

Finish the curry • Once the duck is ready, stir it through the curry sauce • Cook together over a low heat for 5–10 minutes to heat everything through

Finish the rice • After it's been cooking for 10 minutes, remove the pan from the heat and leave the rice to steam for a final 10 minutes, then fluff up the rice with a fork before serving

Time to serve • Trim and thinly slice the spring onions and red chillies • Spoon equal portions of the coconut rice onto 4 serving plates or bowls and serve with the curry • Sprinkle the curry with some Thai basil leaves, red chillies and spring onions before serving

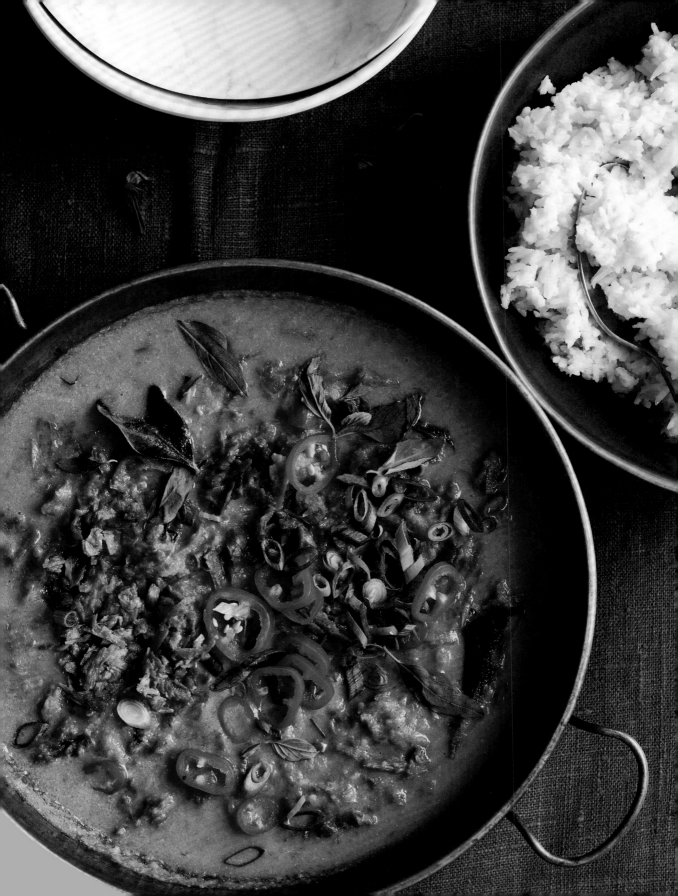

CORONATION CHICKEN SALAD

We've combined oyster mushrooms and plant-based chicken in this recipe for the best pulled texture, and coated it in a creamy dressing made from plant-based mayo, curry powder, mango chutney, turmeric and lime. The mango chutney adds a nice level of sweetness to the sauce, so we've mixed pine nuts through the chicken instead of raisins – for a more classic version, you can mix through raisins if you prefer. Try the salad stuffed in a baguette – it's lush.

SERVES 4

FOR THE CORONATION DRESSING
150g plant-based
    mayonnaise
1 tbsp mild curry powder
2 heaped tbsp
    mango chutney
½ tsp ground turmeric
1 lime
sea salt

FOR THE PULLED CHICKEN
350g oyster mushrooms
2 x 160g packs
    plant-based chicken
2 tbsp olive oil
1 tsp mild curry powder
sea salt

FOR THE SALAD
2 Romaine lettuce hearts
dash of plant-based milk
4 spring onions
1 small bunch of coriander
50g toasted flaked almonds
1 tbsp black sesame seeds
50g pine nuts

Preheat oven to 180°C • Grater • Large baking tray

Make the dressing • In a large mixing bowl, mix together the mayo, curry powder, mango chutney, turmeric and a pinch of salt until smooth • Zest, then halve and juice the lime into the bowl and mix through until smooth

Make the pulled chicken • Using your hands or two forks, tear the oyster mushrooms apart to create a pulled meat-like consistency • Roughly chop the plant-based chicken into small bite-sized pieces • Place the oyster mushrooms and plant-based chicken onto a large baking tray and drizzle with the olive oil, sprinkle with a pinch of salt and add the curry powder • Mix well until the mushrooms and chicken are coated in the oil • Bake in the oven for 30 minutes, stirring halfway through the cooking time

Make the salad • Shred the lettuce leaves widthways until you have a chopped-like consistency • Spoon 4 tablespoons of the dressing into a large mixing bowl and stir through the dash of plant-based milk • Add the shredded lettuce and mix well until all of the leaves are coated in dressing • Trim and slice the spring onions, finely chop the coriander and mix both through the lettuce leaves (saving some to garnish) • Mix through most of the flaked almonds and black sesame seeds (saving some to garnish)

Dress the pulled chicken • Add the cooked pulled oyster mushrooms and chicken to the large bowl along with the dressing and pine nuts • Mix well until all of the pulled mushrooms and plant-based chicken are coated in the dressing

Time to serve • Spoon the dressed leaves onto a large serving plate and use the spoon to spread them out around the entire plate • Pile the dressed chicken high on top of the salad leaves • Top the salad with a sprinkle of the remaining sesame seeds, flaked almonds, chopped coriander and spring onions • Alternatively, stuff it in a roll or baguette (see our sandwich ideas on page 23)

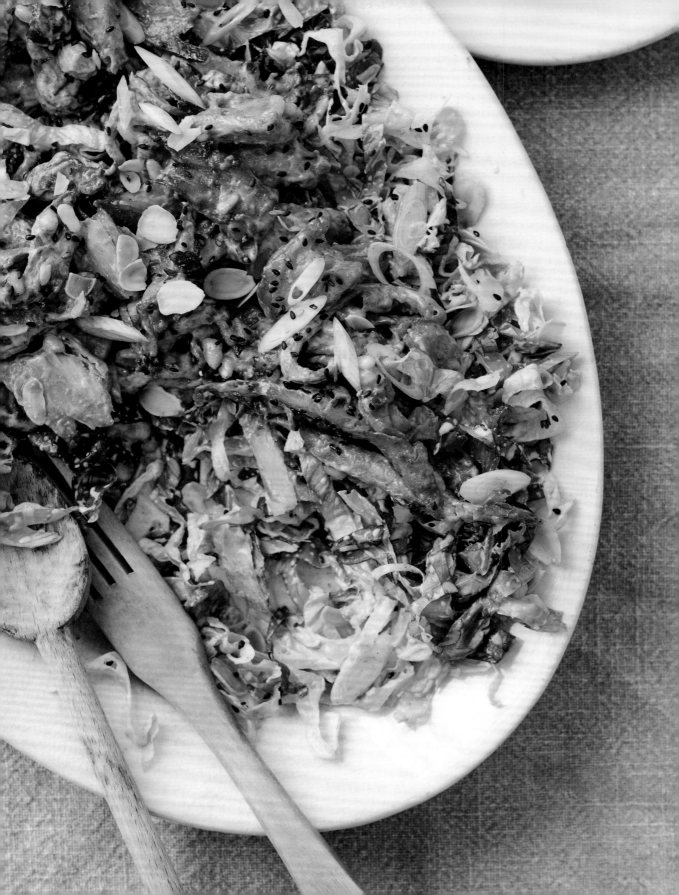

KARE RAISU

Since the late 1800s, curry and rice has been a staple in the Japanese diet. 'Kare raisu' quite simply translates as 'curry rice'. The flavour profile of this dish is very individual, quite different from the curries that hail from India and the surrounding countries. If you like curry but you haven't tried Japanese curry before, we suggest you give this a whirl. We reckon you'll like it.

SERVES 4

FOR THE RICE
480g Japanese short-grain
   rice (sushi rice)
540ml boiling water

FOR THE CURRY ROUX
1 large onion
thumb-sized piece
   of fresh ginger
2 garlic cloves
1 apple
2 tbsp sunflower oil
2 tbsp tomato paste
1 tbsp garam masala
4 tbsp curry powder
3 tbsp plain flour
400ml dry white wine

FOR THE CURRY
2 large carrots
1 large white potato
2 tbsp caster sugar
2 tbsp light soy sauce
2 tbsp ketchup
1 litre boiling water
450g plant-based
   chicken pieces

TO SERVE (OPTIONAL)
fukujinzuke (shop-bought
   Japanese pickles)
chives (for a pop of colour)

Fine grater or microplane • Large saucepan • Medium saucepan and lid

Prepare the rice • Wash the rice in plenty of changes of cold water in a bowl until it starts to run clear • Place the rice back in the bowl, cover with cold water, set to one side and leave to soak for 30 minutes

Prepare the curry roux • Peel and dice the onion • Peel and grate the ginger, garlic and apple • Heat the sunflower oil in a large saucepan over a medium heat, add the onion and cook for 4–5 minutes until translucent • Add the grated ginger, garlic and apple and cook, stirring, for 3–4 minutes • Add the tomato paste and stir for 2 minutes • Add the spices and flour and toast for 2–3 minutes • Add the wine to the pan and turn up the heat to reduce while stirring to avoid any lumps • Cook for 10 minutes

Prepare the vegetables and start the curry • Peel the carrots and potato and cut into 1.5cm pieces, then add them to the roux and stir for 1 minute • Add the sugar, soy sauce and ketchup and cook, stirring, for 1 minute

Finish the curry • Add the litre of boiling water to the curry mixture, bring to a simmer and cook for about 25 minutes until the potatoes are tender and the sauce is well reduced • After 10 minutes add the plant-based chicken

While the curry is simmering, cook the rice • Add the drained, soaked rice and 540ml boiling water to a medium saucepan, put the lid on and cook for 10 minutes over a medium heat • After 10 minutes, as soon as the water has been absorbed, turn off the heat and steam (with the lid on) for 10 minutes (a total of 20 minutes will ensure the rice is cooked properly and perfectly)

Time to serve • Taste the sauce and season to perfection • Spoon the rice into bowls, spoon over the curry, add a little pickle and a few snipped chives (if you like) and serve immediately

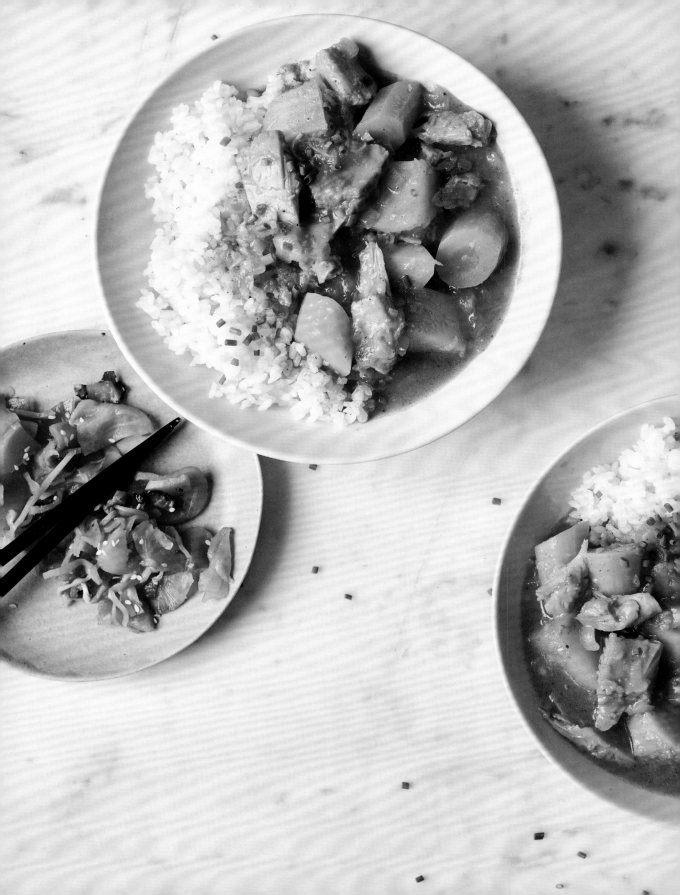

CHICKEN SKEWERS – 3 WAYS

A skewer and a salad is a great option for dinner as it gives you a nice meaty bite and a lovely crispy crunch. We couldn't decide which skewer recipe to include in this book, so we've included three! Teriyaki Skewers with Cucumber Salad for zip and crispness, Souvlaki Skewers with Greek Salad for herbiness and tang and Satay Skewers with Thai Salad for creaminess and crunch.

EACH RECIPE SERVES 2

250g plant-based chicken pieces

FOR THE TERIYAKI MARINADE
4 tsp cornflour
2 tsp water
100ml shop-bought teriyaki marinade
50ml maple syrup

FOR THE CUCUMBER SALAD
½ cucumber
1 garlic clove
25g unsalted peanuts
½ tbsp light soy sauce
½ tbsp rice wine vinegar
½ tbsp toasted sesame oil
½ tsp light brown sugar
½ tsp dried chilli flakes
handful of spring onions
1 tbsp sesame seeds

TERIYAKI SKEWERS WITH CUCUMBER SALAD

2 long skewers – wooden ones will need to be soaked in water for at least 30 minutes • 2 small saucepans • Lasagne dish • Pastry brush

Make the teriyaki marinade • Mix the cornflour and water in a small bowl to form a slurry • Add the teriyaki marinade and maple syrup to a small saucepan and simmer over a medium heat for 3–4 minutes until it starts to thicken • Add the slurry to the pan, reduce the heat and stir until the sauce reaches the consistency of a loose syrup • Transfer the marinade to a bowl and leave to set to the thickness of maple syrup then coat the chicken pieces in the marinade and leave to rest as you make the cucumber salad • Preheat oven to 180°C

Make the cucumber salad • Thinly slice the cucumber widthways • Peel and crush the garlic • Roughly chop the peanuts • Warm another small saucepan over a medium heat, add the garlic and peanuts and toast for a minute until golden and aromatic • Combine the soy sauce, rice wine vinegar, sesame oil, sugar and chilli flakes in a bowl • Add the cucumber and toss until coated • Lay the cucumbers out on a plate • Trim and thinly slice the spring onions and sprinkle them over the cucumber, adding the sesame seeds, garlic and peanuts

Cook the skewers and serve • Pierce the marinated chicken pieces onto skewers and lay them across a lasagne dish to create a makeshift spit – brush any remaining marinade over the pieces • Put the dish in the oven and roast for 13–15 minutes • Take the skewers out of the oven, lay them on the plate with the cucumber and serve immediately

250g plant-based chicken pieces

FOR THE SOUVLAKI MARINADE
1 lemon
handful of fresh parsley
3 tbsp olive oil
1 tbsp tomato purée
½ tbsp dried oregano
½ tbsp smoked paprika
1 tsp ground cumin
1 tsp ground coriander
½ tsp ground black pepper
¼ tsp sea salt

SOUVLAKI SKEWERS WITH GREEK SALAD

2 long skewers – wooden ones will need to be soaked in water for at least 30 minutes • Lasagne dish • Pastry brush

Make the souvlaki marinade • Halve the lemon and chop the parsley • Squeeze the juice from the lemon, catching any pips in your free hand, then combine all the ingredients in a bowl until smooth • Add the chicken pieces, stir to coat in the marinade and set aside • Preheat oven to 180°C

Make the Greek salad • Peel the red onion • Dice the cucumber, tomato and red onion and combine in a bowl • Juice the half lemon into the bowl, catching any pips in your free hand • Transfer the salad to a plate, crumble over the feta and sprinkle over the olives • Combine the rest of the ingredients in a bowl to make a dressing, season with salt and pepper and drizzle over the salad

FOR THE GREEK SALAD
¼ red onion
¼ cucumber
1 tomato
½ lemon
50g plant-based feta
40g kalamata olives
2 tbsp olive oil
½ tsp Dijon mustard
½ tsp dried oregano
sea salt and black pepper

TO GARNISH
fresh dill
fresh parsley

Cook the skewers and serve • Pierce the marinated chicken pieces onto skewers and lay them across a lasagne dish to create a makeshift spit – brush any remaining marinade over the pieces • Put the dish in the oven and roast for 13–15 minutes • Chop the dill and parsley garnish • Take the skewers out of the oven, lay them on the plate with the Greek salad and serve immediately, garnished with the dill and parsley

250g plant-based
   chicken pieces

FOR THE SATAY MARINADE
1 lime
3 tbsp smooth
   peanut butter
1 tbsp light soy sauce
   or tamari
1 tsp plant-based fish
   sauce (optional)
3½ tsp light brown sugar
½ tsp cayenne pepper
   or red chilli powder
   (more to taste)
¼ tsp ground ginger
pinch of ground turmeric
sea salt (if required, the soy
   sauce and peanut butter
   may make it salty enough)

FOR THE THAI SALAD
50g savoy cabbage
1 small carrot (about 50g)
1 spring onion
1 red chilli
5g fresh coriander
1 lime
50g beansprouts
1 tbsp light soy sauce
1 tsp brown sugar
   or maple syrup

TO SERVE
fresh coriander
wedges of lime

SATAY SKEWERS WITH THAI SALAD

2 long skewers – wooden ones will need soaked in water for at least 30 minutes • Small saucepan • Vegetable peeler or mandoline • Lasagne dish • Pastry brush

Make the satay marinade • Halve and juice the lime • Combine all the marinade ingredients in a small saucepan and cook over a low heat until the peanut butter has broken down and the sugar has dissolved • Take the pan off the heat, add the chicken pieces and leave to rest as you make the salad • Preheat oven to 180°C

Make the Thai salad • Finely shred the cabbage and ribbon the carrots using a peeler or mandoline • Trim and thinly slice the spring onion and thinly slice the red chilli • Finely chop the coriander • Halve and juice the lime and mix the juice with the soy sauce and sugar or maple syrup to make a dressing • Combine all the vegetables and herbs on a plate, including the beansprouts, and drizzle the dressing over the salad

Cook the skewers and serve • Pierce the marinated chicken pieces onto skewers and lay them across a lasagne dish to create a makeshift spit – brush any remaining marinade over the pieces • Put the dish in the oven and roast for 13–15 minutes • Take the skewers out of the oven, lay them on the plate with the Thai salad, garnish with coriander and serve immediately with wedges of lime

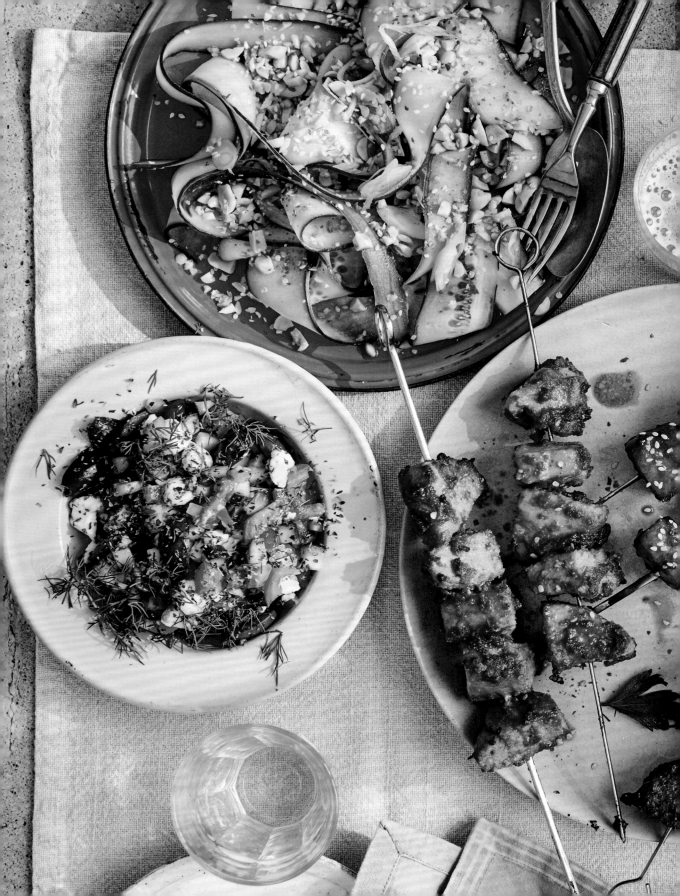

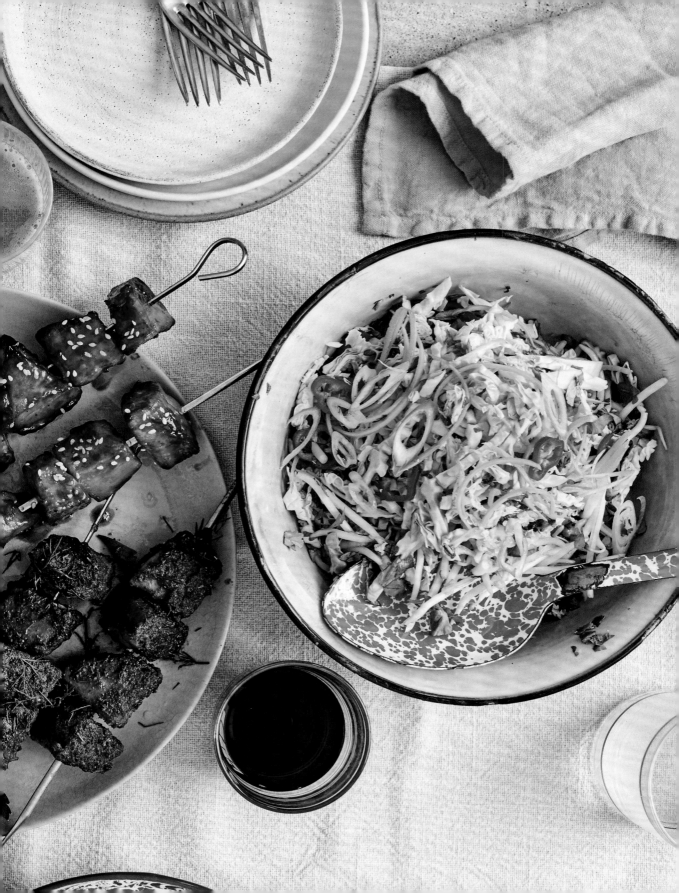

CHICKEN TIKKA MASALA

This is probably the most popular takeaway dish in the UK, so we worked really hard to make this recipe really, really good. It's curiously smoky, pleasantly warming, satisfyingly silky and will blow the tikka masala you get at your local curry house out of the water. Yums, of the highest order.

SERVES 4

**FOR THE
CHICKEN TIKKA**
1 lime
4 garlic cloves
10g fresh ginger
1 tsp sea salt
150ml thick plant-based
    coconut yoghurt
1 tsp ground cumin
1 tsp garam masala
1 tsp smoked sweet paprika
1 tsp ground turmeric
400g plant-based chicken
    pieces

FOR THE SAUCE
1 large onion
10 garlic cloves
10g fresh ginger
1 fresh red chilli
seeds from 1 green
    cardamom pod
3 cinnamon sticks
6 cloves
50g plant-based butter
1 tsp paprika
2 tbsp curry powder
1 x 400g tin chopped
    tomatoes
1 tbsp tomato purée
2 tsp light brown sugar
300ml water
250ml plant-based cream
1 tbsp mango chutney
1 tbsp lemon juice
sea salt

FOR THE RICE
300g basmati rice
600ml cold water
1 tsp fine sea salt

TO SERVE
4 tbsp flaked almonds
10g coriander leaves
8 poppadoms

Fine grater or microplane • Powerful blender • Large frying pan • Small frying pan • Medium saucepan and lid

Marinate the chicken • Halve the lime and squeeze the juice into a mixing bowl • Peel and grate the garlic and ginger and add to the mixing bowl along with the salt, yoghurt and spices • Stir to combine, add the chicken to the bowl, fold into the marinade and set to one side

Prepare the ingredients for the sauce • Peel and thinly slice the onion • Peel the garlic and ginger • Destem and deseed the chilli • Add the cardamom seeds, cinnamon sticks and cloves to a powerful blender, blitz into a powder and transfer to a small bowl • Add the garlic, ginger and chilli to the blender and blitz into a paste

Make the sauce • Add the butter to a large frying pan and melt over a medium heat • Add the sliced onion and a pinch of salt to the pan and fry for 4–5 minutes until soft and golden • Add the paste and cook, stirring, for 2 minutes • Add the powdered spices and stir for 1 minute • Add the tomatoes, tomato purée and sugar to the pan • Add the water to the tin of tomatoes, swill it round, add it to the pan and simmer for 10–12 minutes to reduce • Take the pan off the heat and leave to cool

Cook the rice • Rinse the rice in a sieve under cold running water for 1 minute • Tip into a medium saucepan, pour over the water and sprinkle in the salt • Cover the pan and bring to the boil over a high heat • When the water starts to boil, turn down the heat to low and cook covered for 12 minutes • Take the pan off the heat, keep the lid on and leave to steam • When it's time to serve, remove the lid and fluff up the rice with a fork

Finish the curry • Once the sauce is cool, add to the blender and blitz until smooth • Pour the sauce back into the frying pan and warm to a gentle simmer over a medium heat • Add the paprika and curry powder to the pan and stir into the sauce • Add the cream and mango chutney to the pan and stir into the sauce • Add the marinated chicken (and the marinade), fold into the sauce and simmer for 8 minutes • Add the lemon juice and a little more salt to taste (a touch more mango chutney would work here too)

Time to serve • Toast the flaked almonds in a small dry frying pan over a medium heat for a minute or two, being careful not to let them burn • Spoon the rice into bowls, top with curry, garnish with almonds and fresh coriander and serve immediately with poppadoms

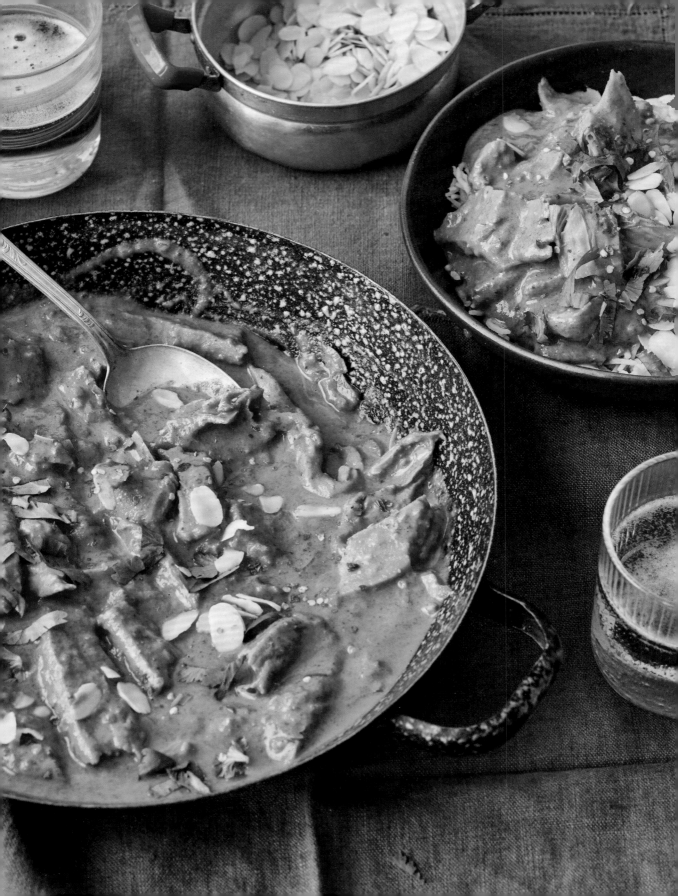

DUCK PANCAKES

Duck pancakes are our favourite starter. In fact, we don't think anything else comes close! Chinese five-spiced jackfruit, roasted until super crispy, then mixed with hoisin sauce and orange juice for the perfect pancake filling. These beauties taste incredible piled up high with crunchy cucumber, spring onions, plum sauce and coriander. The bite of the meat, the sweetness of the sauce, the freshness of the cucumber and spring onion all wrapped up in those delightful thin pancakes. They really are little tubes of heaven that we will NEVER get bored of. Make these, right now. You will not regret it, not one jot.

SERVES 2 FOR MAIN OR 4 FOR STARTER (MAKES 12 PANCAKES)

FOR THE DUCK
1 x 400g tin jackfruit in water, or mock duck
1 tbsp olive oil
1 tbsp toasted sesame oil
1 tbsp chicken seasoning
2 tsp Chinese five-spice
pinch of sea salt

FOR THE PANCAKES
1 medium cucumber
8 spring onions
handful of coriander
12 Chinese pancakes
2 tbsp black and white sesame seeds
6 tbsp plant-based plum sauce

FOR THE SAUCE
1 tbsp tamari
1 heaped tsp shop-bought ginger and garlic paste
1 tbsp toasted sesame oil
4 tbsp hoisin sauce
juice of ½ orange

Preheat oven to 180°C • Large baking tray

First, prepare the duck • Drain and pat-dry the jackfruit, then place into a large baking tray and shred using two forks until it has a pulled-like consistency (remove any seeds – they look a little like cannellini beans) • Add the olive oil, toasted sesame oil, chicken seasoning, Chinese five-spice and salt • Mix well until all of the jackfruit is coated in the oil and roast in the oven for 30–35 minutes until cooked and crispy, tossing halfway through to ensure they are cooked evenly

Prepare the rest of the ingredients • Trim and halve the cucumber lengthways then scoop out the seeds with a spoon • Cut the two long halves into thirds and cut the thirds into fine matchsticks • Trim and halve the spring onions lengthways, then cut into pieces the same length as the cucumber pieces • Chop the coriander

Cook the pancakes • Cook the Chinese pancakes according to the packet instructions

Make the sauce • Mix the sauce ingredients together in a small bowl until smooth

Finish the duck • Once cooked, take the jackfruit out of the oven and mix through the sauce, ensuring all of the jackfruit is coated

Time to serve • Transfer the duck to a serving bowl • Transfer the prepared veggies to serving bowls and put the bowls on the table • Lay the duck, spring onions, cucumber, sesame seeds and coriander on top of the pancakes, drizzle over some plum sauce. Roll the pancakes up neatly and enjoy!

NOTE
You can also use 600g king oyster mushrooms in this recipe – simply swap them for the jackfruit and follow the same instructions.

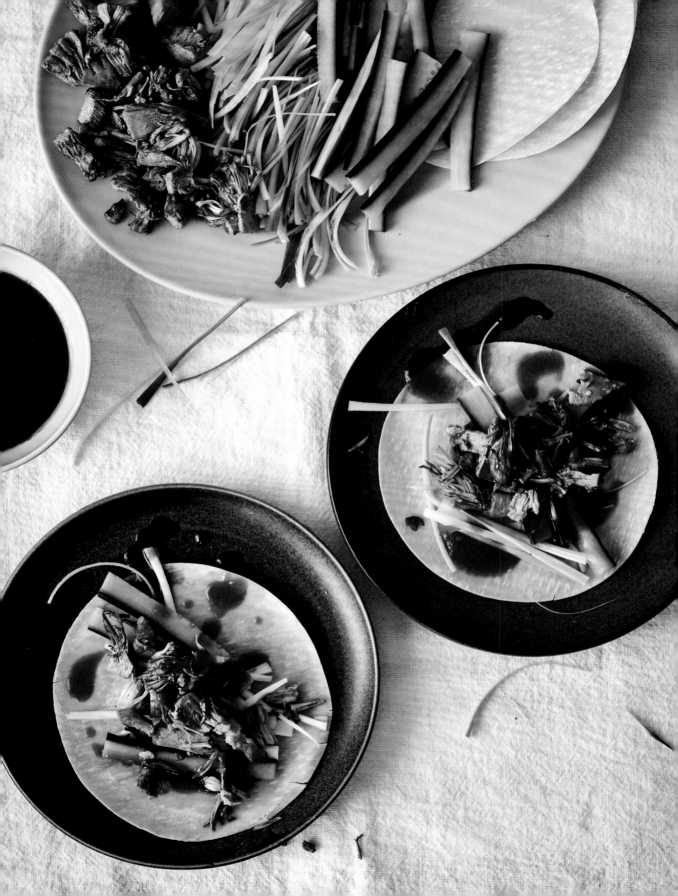

KUNG PAO CHICKEN

A little spice, a little sweetness, a bit of bite that's just like meat. This is fantastic fakeaway food for anyone who likes a little bit of kick. Serve it on its own with rice during the week, or make a couple more dishes for a wonderful Friday-night spread.

SERVES 2

FOR THE CHICKEN MARINADE
1 tbsp toasted sesame oil
2 tsp light soy sauce
1 tbsp maple syrup
1 tbsp cornflour
¼–½ tsp cayenne pepper
320g plant-based
    chicken pieces

FOR THE RICE
150g basmati rice
300ml cold water
½ tsp fine sea salt

FOR THE SAUCE AND VEGETABLES
2.5cm piece of fresh ginger
2 garlic cloves
200g red and/or orange
    peppers
2 spring onions
2 tbsp toasted sesame oil
50g unsalted peanuts
2 tbsp cornflour plus
    2 tbsp water
2 tbsp light soy sauce
1 tbsp light brown sugar
    or maple syrup (or
    more to taste)
1 tbsp Shaoxing rice wine
½ tsp red chilli powder (or
    more if you like it spicy)
½ tsp ground black pepper
200ml vegetable stock
sea salt

TO SERVE
20g unsalted peanuts
1 spring onion

Medium saucepan • Wok or frying pan • 2 medium frying pans

Prepare the kung pao chicken • Mix all the marinade ingredients in a medium bowl • Coat the chicken pieces in the marinade and set aside for at least 30 minutes

Cook the rice • Rinse the rice in a sieve under cold running water for 1 minute • Tip into a medium saucepan, pour over the water and the salt • Cover the pan and bring to the boil over a high heat • When the water starts to boil, turn down the heat to low and cook covered for 12 minutes • Take the pan off the heat, keep the lid on and leave to steam

Make the kung pao sauce • Peel and finely dice the ginger and garlic • Halve, core and dice the peppers into 1.5cm pieces • Trim and cut the spring onions into 1cm pieces • Heat 1 tablespoon of the sesame oil in a wok or frying pan over a low heat, then add the peanuts and cook for 1–2 minutes until lightly browned • Add the ginger and garlic and cook for 1–2 minutes until soft and fragrant • Add the peppers and cook for 2 minutes • Mix the cornflour with the water in a small glass then add to the wok • Add the soy sauce, sugar, rice wine, chilli powder, ground black pepper, vegetable stock and a pinch of salt and stir to combine • Reduce the heat to a very gentle simmer

Cook the kung pao chicken • Warm the remaining sesame oil in a medium frying pan over a high heat • Add the marinated chicken to the frying pan and fry for 3–4 minutes until the chicken is developing a crisp edge (or however long it states on the chicken packet)

Combine the elements • Crush the peanuts (to serve) • Loosen the sauce with a little water if it appears too thick • Add the spring onions and chicken to the pan and fold into the sauce

Time to serve • Trim and thinly slice the spring onion • Spoon the rice into bowls, top with kung pao chicken, garnish with sliced spring onion and crushed peanuts and serve immediately

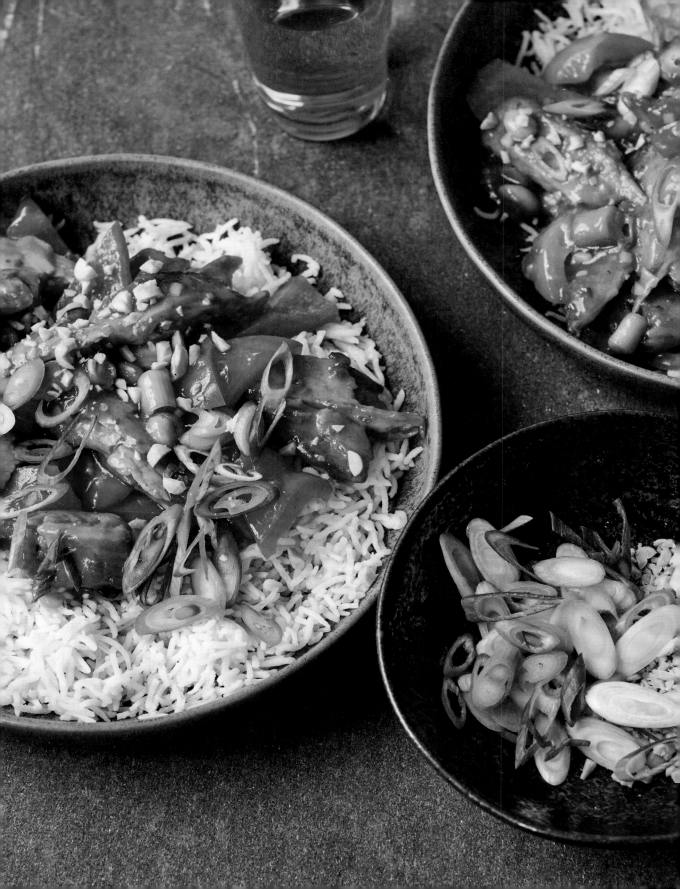

KO CLUB SANDWICH

Club sandwiches might be the most popular sandwiches in the world and it's easy to see why. Perfectly seasoned chicken and smoky sweet bacon complemented with crunchy lettuce, silky mayo and juicy tomato all wrapped up in crispy golden toast. Served with French fries or a bag of crisps and an ice-cold coke, this is a real knock-out lunch.

MAKES 2 CLUB SANDWICHES

FOR THE CHICKEN
3 fat king oyster mushrooms
2 tbsp olive oil
1 tbsp chicken seasoning
1 tsp dried sage
sea salt and black pepper

FOR THE MUSHROOM BACON AND MARINADE
2 tbsp olive oil
1 tbsp maple syrup
1 tbsp tamari
1 tsp smoked paprika
½ tsp garlic powder
1 tsp liquid smoke (optional)
2 king oyster mushrooms

FOR THE SANDWICHES
1 vine-ripened tomato
1 small romaine lettuce
6 slices of thick white bread
4 tbsp plant-based mayonnaise
8 toothpicks

TO SERVE
a large bag of crisps

Preheat oven to 190°C • Baking tray lined with baking parchment • Large frying pan • Toaster or grill

Prepare the chicken • Cut the caps off the king oyster mushrooms and save them for another recipe • Roughly tear the mushroom stems into strips about 1cm thick • Put the mushroom strips in a bowl, drizzle with the olive oil and sprinkle over the chicken seasoning, sage and a little salt and pepper • Toss to combine, making sure the mushrooms are well coated

Cook the chicken • Spread the mushrooms out on a lined baking tray, making sure they are evenly spaced out • Place the tray in the oven and cook for 25–30 minutes, or until golden

Make the marinade for the mushroom bacon • Put all the marinade ingredients (except for the mushrooms) in a large mixing bowl and stir well to combine

Prepare the mushroom bacon • Cut the caps off the king oyster mushrooms and save them for another recipe • Slice the mushrooms lengthways into 5mm-thick slices • Add all of the strips to the marinade bowl • Toss well to coat all of the strips in the liquid and leave to marinate for at least 10 minutes

Prepare the remaining ingredients • Thinly slice the tomato • Cut the lettuce lengthways in half, cut out the white core and roughly shred the leaves • Toast the bread

Fry the mushroom bacon • Place a large frying pan over a medium heat • Once warm, lay the marinated mushroom bacon strips in the frying pan and fry over a medium-high heat for 5–6 minutes, turning halfway through

Build the sandwiches • Lay 2 slices of toast down on a chopping board and spread 1 tablespoon of the mayo over each • Top each slice with shredded lettuce, then with strips of the chicken • Top the chicken with another slice of toast • Spread each slice of toast with another tablespoon of mayo • Top both with sliced tomato, then with strips of the mushroom bacon • Top the sandwiches with the remaining toast

Time to serve • Push 4 toothpicks into each sandwich, 2.5cm in from each corner • Cut the sandwiches into 4 triangles, plate up and serve straight away with crisps

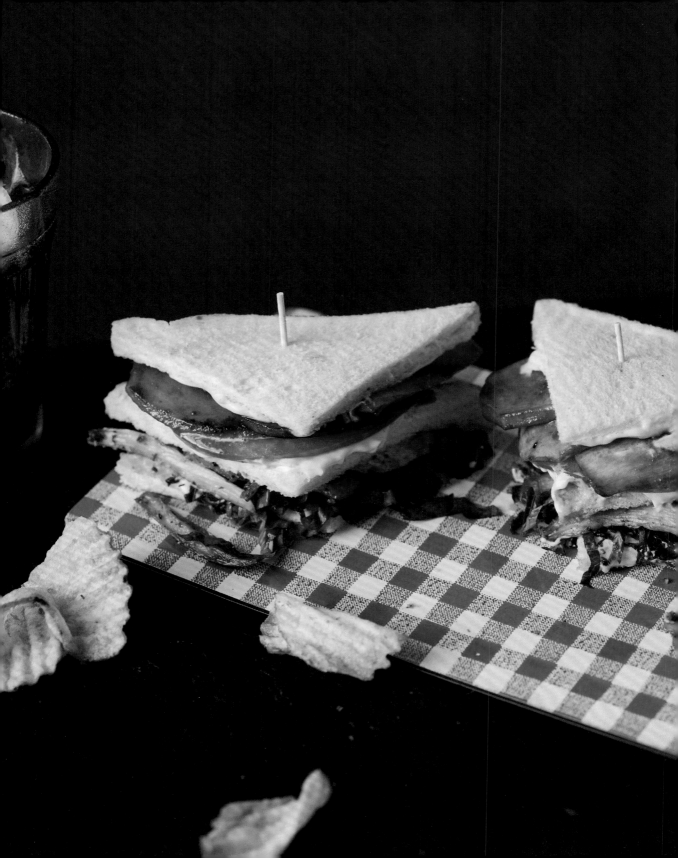

BEEF

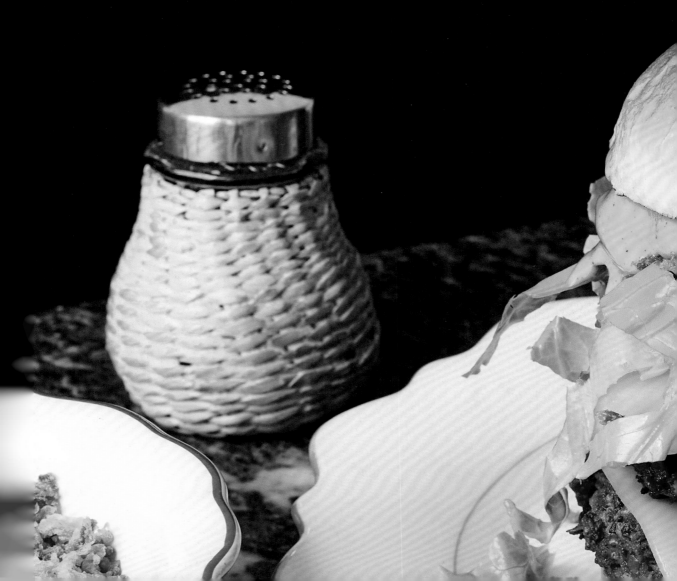

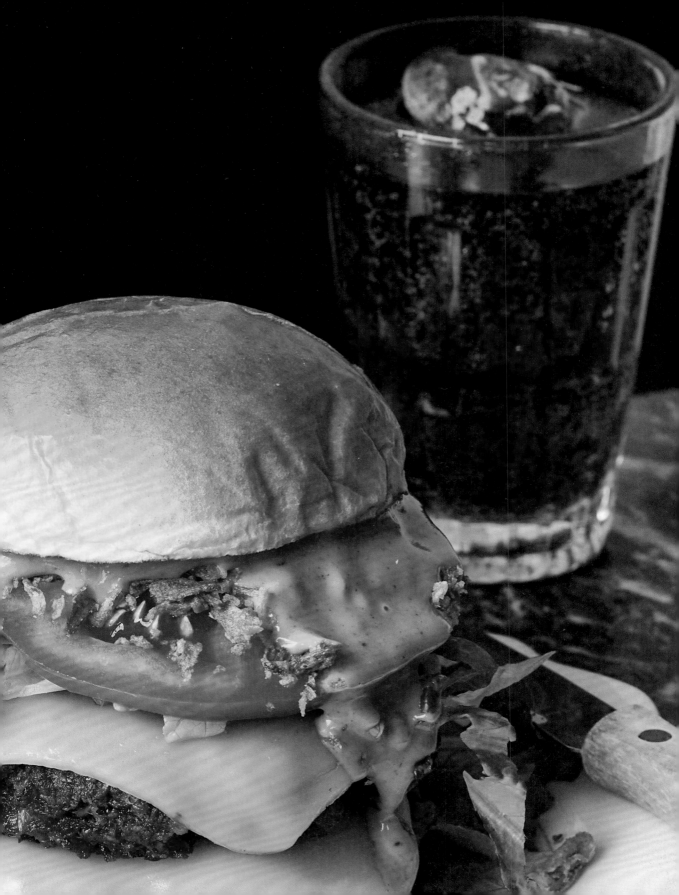

PHILLY CHEESESTEAK

VisitPhilly.com states that; 'In 1930, the cheesesteak was invented when Pat Olivieri, a hot dog vendor and namesake to Pat's King of Steaks, threw beef on his grill to make a sandwich.' Our version is certainly a little different to Pat's, but we're pretty sure that if he tried this one, he'd be mighty impressed.

SERVES 4

3 white onions
45ml sunflower oil
1 tbsp cider vinegar
300g chestnut mushrooms
1 green pepper
2 plant-based OXO cubes
380ml boiling water
4 plant-based steaks
   (soy/pea protein)
4 plant-based brioche
   hot-dog rolls
25g plant-based butter
150g grated white plant-
   based cheese (we used
   plant-based mozzarella)
sea salt and black pepper

TO SERVE
8 large pickled gherkins
American mustard, to taste

Preheat oven to 180°C • Large saucepan with lid • Large frying pan • Heatproof jug • Large baking sheet • Tongs

Prepare and cook the onions • Peel and slice the onions 'Lyonnaise style' (cut in half, remove the root and tip, and slice thinly with the knife passing through base and top rather than across the onion) • Warm half the oil in a large saucepan over a medium heat, add the onions and a pinch of salt, stir to coat, put the lid on and leave the onions to steam for 3–4 minutes • Take the lid off and fry over a medium-low heat for 5–6 minutes, stirring occasionally, until golden, sticky and sweet • Add the vinegar to the pan and stir to deglaze

Prepare and cook the mushrooms • De-stem and slice the mushrooms • Halve, core and thinly slice the green pepper • Warm some of the remaining oil in a large frying pan over a medium heat • Add the mushrooms to the pan with a pinch each of salt and pepper and fry for 5–10 minutes until golden and fragrant • Add the green pepper to the pan after 3–4 minutes • Once cooked, add the mushroom mixture to the onions, stir to combine and set to one side • Don't clean out the mushroom pan

Prepare and cook the steak • Crumble the OXO cubes into a heatproof jug and cover with the boiling water • Transfer a third of the stock to a mug and set to one side • Pour the remaining two-thirds of the stock in the pan containing the mushrooms, onion and green pepper mixture • Slice the steaks on an angle to make a slightly larger surface area • Warm a splash of oil in the pan you fried the mushrooms in over a medium heat, add the slices of steak and fry for a couple of minutes • Add the stock from the mug and simmer the steak over a medium-high heat for a few minutes until most of the stock has reduced • Pour the mushroom, onion and green pepper mixture into the pan containing the steak and reduce until nearly all the moisture has evaporated • Taste and season to perfection

Time to serve • Slice the hot-dog rolls, spread with butter and toast in the oven on a baking sheet for 3–4 minutes until slightly crisp • Plate up the rolls, use tongs to fill the hoagies with the steak filling, top with the cheese and serve immediately with gherkins and American mustard

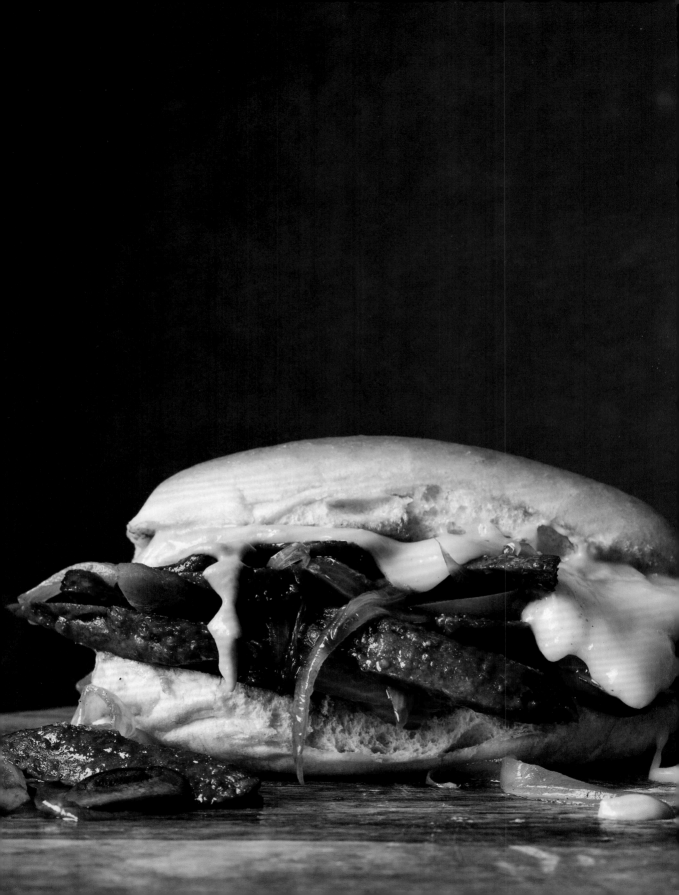

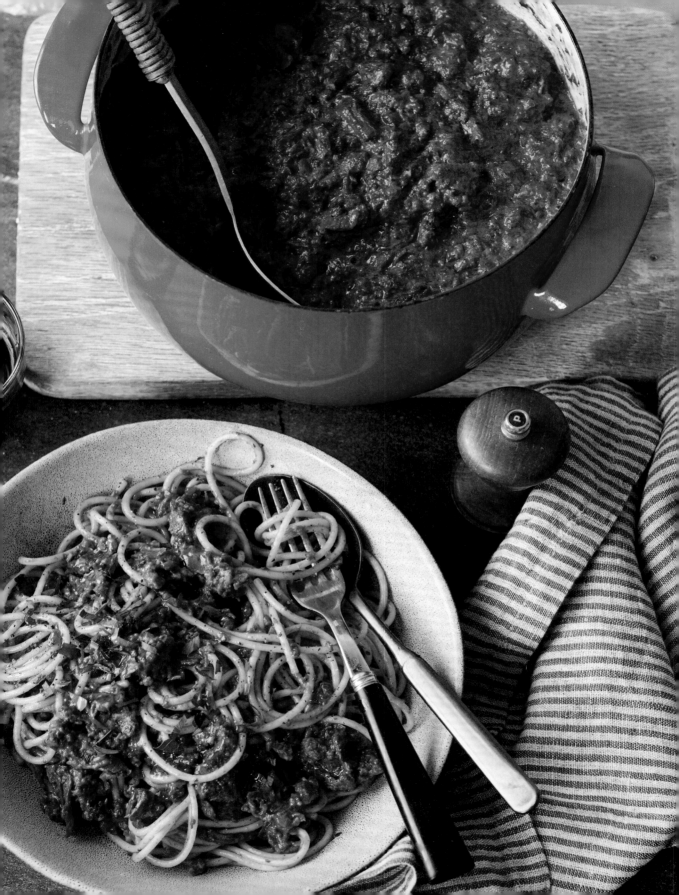

ULTIMATE BOLOGNESE

We've written a fair few bolognese recipes in our time, but this one is the ultimate. Rich, deep and complex, you might as well fold the corner of this page because you'll visit this recipe time and time again. Serve it over pasta, in a lasagne, on top of polenta or in pastry. Either way, it'll put a smile on your face.

SERVES 8

FOR THE MINCE
150g plant-based bacon
800g chestnut mushrooms
300g plant-based mince
1 tsp salt
1 tsp ground black pepper
75ml olive oil

FOR THE SAUCE
1 onion
8 garlic cloves
2 carrots
10g thyme sprigs
½ fennel bulb
2 celery sticks
50ml olive oil
2 tsp sea salt
1 tsp dried chilli flakes
375ml plant-based red wine
1 x 400g tin plum tomatoes
100g dried porcini
    mushrooms, soaked
    according to packet
    instructions then drained
1 tbsp light brown sugar
3 tbsp Henderson's relish
100g tomato purée
100ml plant-based cream
sea salt and black pepper

Food processor • Large sauté pan

Prepare the mince ingredients • Roughly slice the bacon and mushrooms • Add them to a food processor with the plant-based mince, salt and pepper and pulse into a mince (you may need to do this in batches, depending on the size of your processor bowl)

Prepare the mince • Heat the 75ml olive oil in a large sauté pan over a medium-high heat • Roll the mince mixture into walnut-sized balls, flatten them into patties and fry in the pan in batches for a couple of minutes on each side to brown slightly • Set the patties to one side • This will ensure that the texture of the mince is perfect

Prepare the remaining ingredients • Peel and roughly chop the onion, garlic and carrots • Pick the thyme leaves by running your fingers and thumbs down the stalks • Trim and roughly chop the fennel • Trim and cut the celery into chunks • Add all the ingredients to the food processor (it doesn't have to be clean) and pulse until diced

Cook the bolognese • Heat the 50ml olive oil in the large sauté pan over a medium-high heat • Add the onion mixture to the pan with the salt and the chilli flakes and fry for 8–10 minutes, stirring occasionally, until soft and golden • Pour the red wine into the pan to deglaze and simmer for 5–7 minutes • Add the patties to the pan and stir for 2 minutes • Add the plum tomatoes, dried mushrooms, brown sugar, Henderson's relish and tomato purée to the pan and stir to combine • Cook the bolognese for 25–30 minutes, stirring occasionally to prevent it catching and adding a splash of water if it seems too thick

Time to serve • Pour the plant-based cream into the pan and stir it into the sauce • Taste, season to perfection and serve with rice, polenta, rice, mash or our favourite, pasta!

CHILLI CHEESEBURGER NACHOS

Nancy Sinatra's boots were made for walking, but our Chilli Cheeseburger Nachos were made for sharing. This is THE recipe to make if you've got a bunch of buddies coming round to yours to watch the footy. Now, come on you blues! (or reds, if you're that way inclined).

SERVES 4–6

FOR THE CHEESE SAUCE
150g white potato
100g sweet potato
40g raw unsalted cashews
10g nooch (nutritional yeast)
1 tsp paprika
1 tsp onion powder
1 tsp garlic powder
sea salt

FOR THE BURGER SAUCE
120g plant-based mayonnaise
60g ketchup
2 tsp gherkin pickle juice
1 tsp ground black pepper

FOR THE BURGER PATTIES
20ml olive oil
4 plant-based burger patties
2–3 tbsp juice from the jar of jalapeños

TO SERVE
¼ iceberg lettuce
1 beef tomato
3 large pickled gherkins
200g plant-based cheddar
100g pickled sliced jalapeños
350g corn tortilla chips (we like to use Xochitl or Manomasa chips)
40g crispy fried onions

2 medium saucepans • Jug blender • Box grater • Frying pan • Deep oven tray

Prepare the cheese sauce • Peel the two types of potatoes and cut into small dice • Bring a saucepan of salted water to the boil over a high heat • Add the cubed potatoes to the pan and cook for 12 minutes until tender • Add the cashews to a second saucepan of boiling water and simmer for 10–12 minutes • Drain the tender potatoes but reserve the water • Drain the cashews and add them to a jug blender along with the cooked potatoes, nooch, paprika, onion powder and garlic powder • Blitz until completely smooth, adding some reserved potato water if you need to thin it out a little – the yield will be 750–800g • Set to one side

Prepare the burger sauce • Put the mayo, ketchup, gherkin juice and ground black pepper in a bowl and stir to combine • Put the bowl in the fridge and save till later

Prepare the serving ingredients • Shred the lettuce • Dice the beef tomato • Slice the gherkins • Grate the cheese

Prepare the burger patties • Heat the oil in a frying pan over a medium heat and fry the burgers for 3 minutes on one side • Flip the burgers and fry for a couple of minutes on the other side then add the 2–3 tablespoons of jalapeño pickle juice from the jar and switch off the heat • Remove the burgers from the pan, place them on a chopping board and leave to rest for a few minutes before cutting them into small pieces • Preheat oven to 180°C

Assemble the nachos • Cover the base of a deep oven tray with tortilla chips, sprinkle over some burger pieces, jalapeños, tomato, cheddar, gherkins, crispy fried onions and drizzle over some cheese sauce • Repeat until all the ingredients have been added to the tray in layers (reserve a few tomato slices, crispy onions and gherkins for the top) • Put the tray the oven and roast for 3–4 minutes

Time to serve • Remove the tray from the oven, sprinkle over the lettuce and reserved tomatoes, crispy fried onions and gherkins • Drizzle over the burger sauce and serve immediately with a few cold beers

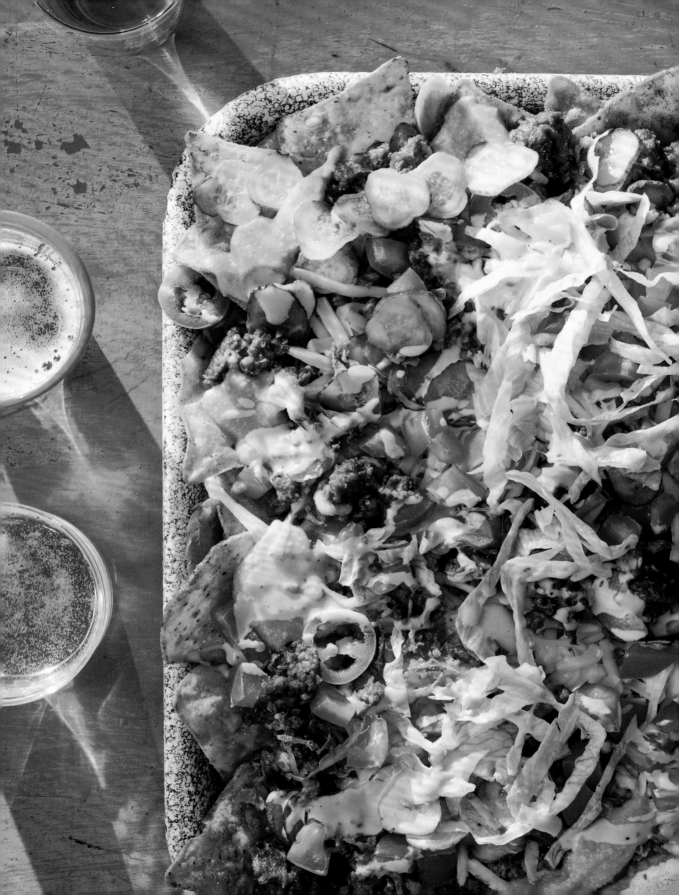

ORZO MEATBALLS

Orzo – a type of pasta – is an ingredient we don't use very often but when we do use it, we're always left wondering why we don't use it more often because it's lovely. On the subject of lovely, the inspiration for this magnificent recipe came from the queen of cooking herself, Nigella Lawson.

SERVES 4

FOR THE MEATBALLS
20g flat-leaf parsley
    (including the stalks)
3 garlic cloves
2 tbsp chia seeds
600g plant-based mince
3 tbsp panko breadcrumbs
4 tbsp nooch (nutritional
    yeast) or grated plant-
    based parmesan
2 tsp sea salt
2 tsp ground black pepper

FOR THE SAUCE
1 small onion
20ml olive oil
1 tsp sea salt flakes
250ml plant-based
    white wine
2 x 400g tins chopped
    tomatoes
3 tbsp tomato purée
1 tsp paprika
½ tsp dried chilli flakes
1 tbsp red wine vinegar
1 tbsp light brown sugar
2 tbsp plant-based butter
285ml cold water
250g orzo pasta

TO SERVE
handful of fresh parsley
sprinkle of nooch
    (nutritional yeast) or
    plant-based parmesan
small bag of fresh rocket
squeeze of lemon juice

Large heavy-based saucepan with lid

Make the meatball mixture • Finely chop the parsley and set aside • Peel and finely chop the garlic • Soak the chia seeds in a bowl with 4 tablespoons of cold water for about 10 minutes until it forms a gel • Place all the ingredients for the meatballs into a large bowl and mix together with your hands, being sure not to overmix, as it will make the meatballs dense-textured and heavy

Make the meatballs • Pinch out pieces of the mix and form them into walnut-size balls, putting them on a clean plate as you go • You should get about 20 meatballs

Make the sauce • Peel and finely dice the onion • Heat the oil in a heavy-based saucepan that's large enough to take the meatballs and pasta • Add the chopped onion with the salt and cook over a medium heat, stirring every now and again, for about 10 minutes until softened • Add the wine and simmer for a further 10 minutes • Add the tomatoes, tomato purée, paprika, chilli flakes, vinegar, brown sugar and butter • Fill both the empty tins with the water, give them a good swill, pour into the pan, bring the sauce to a simmer, put the lid on and cook for 30–35 minutes

Cook the meatballs • Drop the meatballs gently into the simmering sauce • Bring back to the boil, turn the heat down again to a simmer, put the lid back on and simmer the meatballs for 15 minutes

Add the pasta • Tip in the orzo, stir gently and increase the heat to bring the mixture back to a bubble • Simmer for 15 minutes, or until the pasta is cooked • You will have to stir it occasionally throughout this time to make sure the orzo isn't sticking to the bottom of the pan

Time to serve • Chop the parsley (to serve) • Spoon the pasta into bowls, sprinkle with parsley, nooch and a handful of rocket, add a squeeze of lemon juice and tuck in

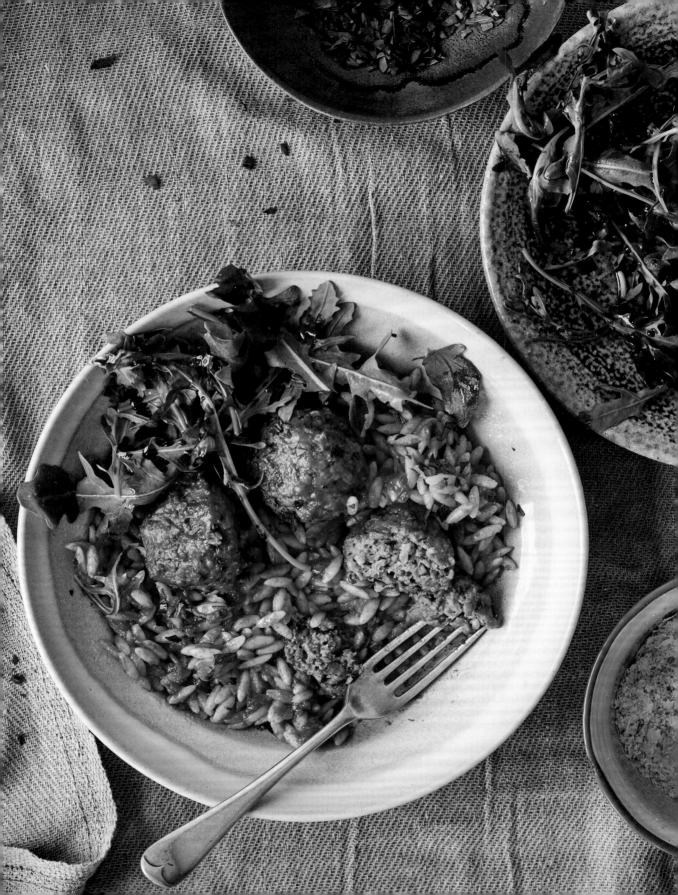

KEEMA PARATHA WITH COCONUT CHUTNEY

We've taken inspiration from the best of North Indian and South Indian food in this dish of pillowy bread stuffed with succulent spicy mince. Sounds good, right? You can eat this on its own a bit like a sandwich, but you can also serve it with a nice saucy curry in place of naan bread. Rip it, dip it and get stuck right in!

SERVES 4–6

FOR THE PARATHA DOUGH

500g plain flour, plus extra for dusting
2 tsp sea salt
4 tsp nigella seeds
120g coconut yoghurt
about 100ml lukewarm water

FOR THE MINCE

½ onion
4 green bird's-eye chillies
50g fresh coriander (leaves and stalks)
2cm piece of fresh ginger
4 garlic cloves
20g fresh mint
2 tbsp vegetable oil
1 tbsp garam masala
1 tbsp ground cumin
½ tsp asafoetida
1 tbsp ground coriander
1½ tsp ground turmeric
1 tbsp nooch (nutritional yeast)
300g plant-based mince
115ml water
150g petits pois
½ tsp sea salt
½ lime

FOR THE COCONUT CHUTNEY

100g desiccated coconut
50ml lukewarm water
4 spring onions
1 fresh green chilli
1 garlic clove
1 small shallot
80g fresh mint
2 limes
120g coconut yoghurt
80ml rapeseed oil
1 tsp sea salt

TO SERVE

plant-based butter
fresh coriander

Fine grater or microplane • Heavy-based saucepan • Food processor • Rolling pin • Griddle pan or frying pan • Pastry brush

Make the paratha dough • Put the flour, salt, nigella seeds and yoghurt in a large bowl and mix with your hands to make a crumbly mixture • Add splashes of water little by little and knead to make a soft dough • Cover the bowl with a damp cloth or tea towel and set aside for 20–30 minutes while you make the filling

Prepare the vegetables for the filling • Peel and finely dice the onion • Thinly slice the chillies • Thinly slice the coriander stalks • Peel and grate the ginger and garlic • Pick the mint leaves and thinly slice

Prepare the filling • Heat the vegetable oil in a heavy-based saucepan over a medium heat • Add the onion and a pinch of salt and fry for 3 minutes, stirring frequently, until translucent • Add the ginger, garlic, coriander stalks and chillies and stir-fry for 2 minutes • Add the ground spices and nooch and stir to combine • Add the plant-based mince and water, stir and leave to cook for 12 minutes until almost all the water has been absorbed • Take the pan off the heat and stir in the peas, salt, mint and coriander leaves • Squeeze in the lime juice • Take the pan off the heat and leave to cool to room temperature • Add the mixture to a food processor and pulse until coarsely mixed • Transfer the mixture to a bowl and wash out the processor

Make the chutney • Soak the desiccated coconut in the water and set aside • Trim the spring onions and cut into chunks • Destem, deseed and roughly chop the chilli • Peel the garlic and small shallot • Pick the mint leaves • Halve the limes and squeeze the juice into the food processor • Add the rest of the chutney ingredients and blitz to form a textured purée

Build the paratha • Divide the dough into 8 equal pieces • Dust the balls with a little flour and roll out to make a 10cm circle • Add about 65g of filling mixture into the centre of the dough and bring the edges together to cocoon the filling • Dust with flour and gently roll the balls into a 13–15cm circle • Heat a griddle pan or dry frying pan over a medium-high heat and melt some butter in a saucepan • Place a paratha on the hot griddle and cook for about 4 minutes, using a flat spatula to apply pressure and flip them every minute or so and brushing the paratha with melted butter as they cook until golden, shiny, flaky and cooked through

Time to serve • Finely chop the coriander • Transfer the paratha onto a plate, sprinkle over a little coriander and serve immediately with the coconut chutney

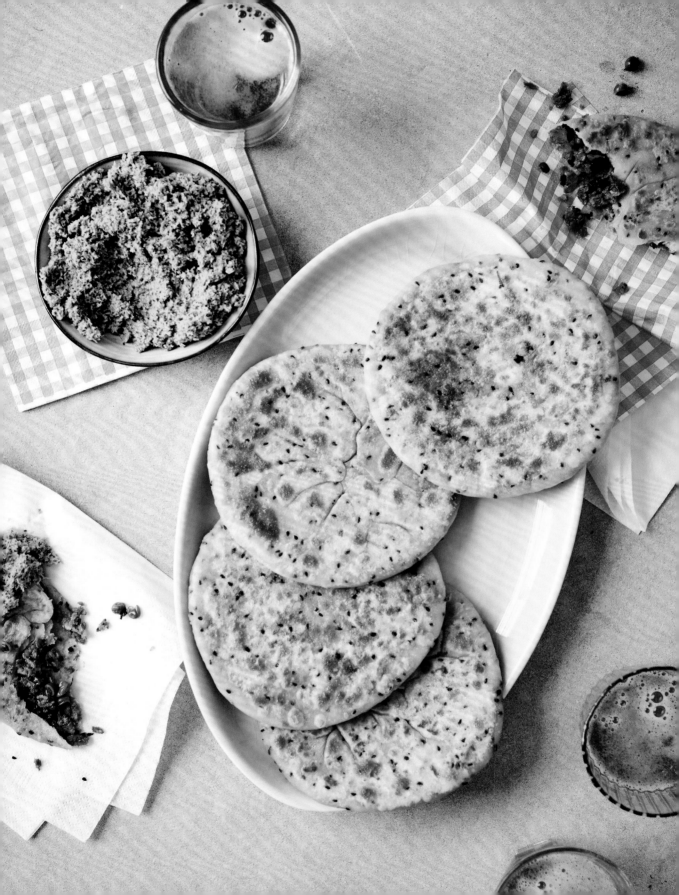

CARNE ASADA TACOS

We LOVE tacos, they're such a treat. They're pretty much the perfect food for a casual social occasion. A few drinks, a bit of sunshine, some mates, lots of chat, plenty of laughs and a few tacos. You can't go wrong really, can you! In fact, our good friend Joe runs a mezcal bar-come-tacoria called PINA in the Kelham Island area of Sheffield. Their cocktails are as good as any you'll find anywhere, and their vegan menu is jam-packed with delicious tacos that you just won't be able to say no to.

Anyway, as you've probably worked out, we love tacos and if you cook this recipe at home, we reckon you'll end up loving them too!

SERVES 4

600g plant-based steak

FOR THE MARINADE
8g fresh coriander
4 garlic cloves
1 big orange
1 big lemon
2 limes
60ml sunflower oil
60ml light soy sauce
½ tsp ground cumin
½ tsp smoked paprika
½ tsp ground black pepper
1 tsp chopped chipotle in
    adobo or adobe paste
½ tsp chilli powder
½ tsp dried oregano
generous pinch of salt

FOR THE GUACAMOLE
3 ripe avocados
2 or 3 limes
1 echalion shallot
2 red chillies
1 garlic clove
15g fresh coriander
sea salt

Fine grater or microplane • Balloon whisk • Sealable container • Medium saucepan • Griddle pan • Tongs • Frying pan

Make the marinade • Pick the coriander leaves and shred • Peel and grate the garlic • Halve and juice the citrus fruits • Add all the marinade ingredients to a bowl and stir with a balloon whisk or fork

Prepare and marinate the steak • Slice the plant-based steak into 1cm-thick strips, lay them into a sealable container, cover with half the marinade, put the lid on, give it a shake and leave to marinate • Set the remaining marinade to one side

Prepare the red onion to serve • Peel and finely dice the red onion, put it in a bowl and cover with cold water (this will soften the flavour)

Prepare the guacamole • Halve, destone and scoop the avocado out of the skins • Place half the avocado in a bowl and mash it with the back of a fork • Cut the remaining avocado into 5mm chunks • Halve the limes • Peel and finely dice the shallot • Halve, deseed and dice the chillies • Peel and grate the garlic • Rip the coriander leaves away from the stalks and thinly slice the leaves • Squeeze the lime juice into the bowl, add the shallot, chilli, garlic and coriander leaves to the bowl and stir to combine • Taste the guacamole and season with salt • Fold in the remaining avocado chunks and set to one side

Cook the steak • Pour the reserved marinade and the marinade from the steak container into a medium saucepan and simmer over a medium heat until reduced by half • Warm a griddle pan over a medium heat, tip the steak strips onto the pan and sizzle, turning them occasionally, for 3–4 minutes • Transfer the griddled steak into the saucepan, stir to coat and turn the heat down to low

TO SERVE
½ red onion
8–12 corn tacos
2 limes
60g plant-based feta
extra coriander leaves
    (optional)
hot sauce (optional)

Prepare the tacos • Warm a dry frying pan over a medium heat and toast the tacos individually for 10 seconds on each side • Stack them on a plate and cover with a clean cloth

Time to serve • Cut the limes into wedges • Crumble the plant-based feta into a bowl • Drain the red onion with a sieve, squeezing out excess water with the back of a spoon and place them in a bowl • Transfer the steak and guacamole to bowls • Take all the elements to the table with a few cold beers, let all your guests build their own and tuck in!

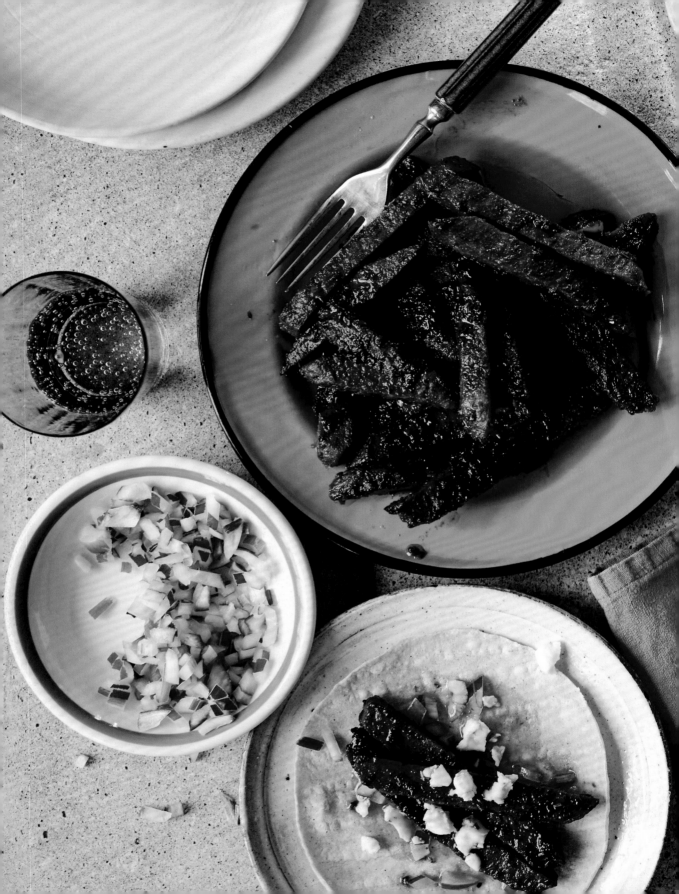

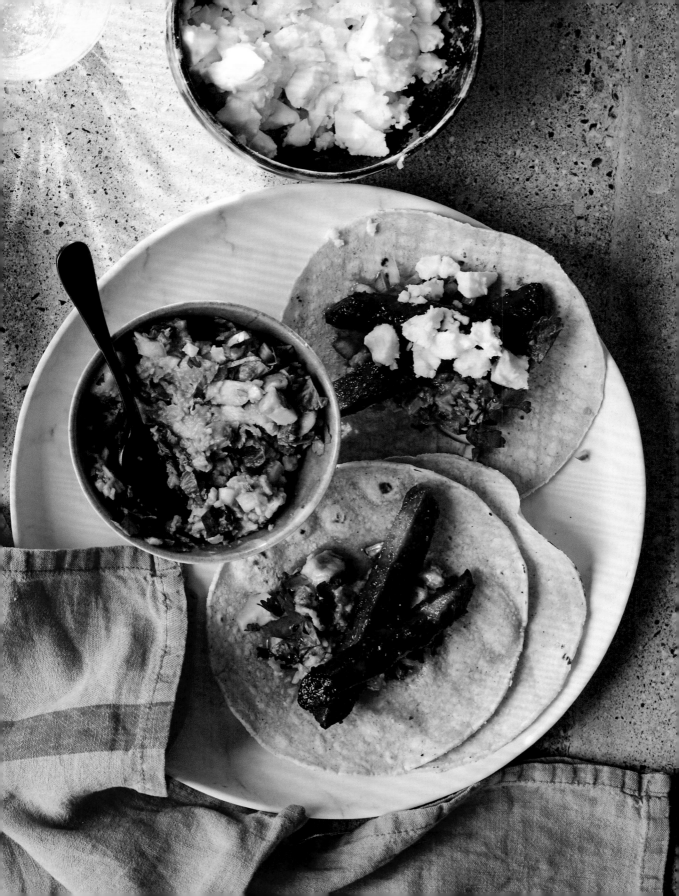

BOEUF BOURGUIGNON

If you're reading this between the months of October and March, we urge you to make this Bourguignon. It's warming, hearty and bursting with flavour. The boeuf bourguignon sauce is rich and wholesome, packed with red wine and fruity flavours, and simmered down in a low oven until perfect. We serve it with the silkiest mash in the world, pushed through a sieve to create the perfect consistency, but you could quite easily use buttery new potatoes, creamy polenta or mafaldine pasta. Stews really don't come much better than this – enjoy!

SERVES 4

FOR THE BOEUF BOURGUIGNON
2 onions
3 garlic cloves
2 carrots
splash of olive oil
2 x 227g packs plant-based steak pieces
150g plant-based bacon lardons (or plant-based bacon cut into small pieces)
150g button mushrooms
120g pickled pearl onions
3 tbsp tomato purée
1 vegetable stock pot
300ml boiling water
400ml plant-based red wine (mild flavoured)
3 fresh thyme or rosemary sprigs
2 large bay leaves (or 3 small)
2 tsp tamari
2 tsp light brown sugar
sea salt and black pepper

FOR THE MASHED POTATO
1kg Maris Piper potatoes
100g plant-based butter
4 tbsp plant-based milk, plus more if needed
sea salt and black pepper

TO SERVE (OPTIONAL)
handful of parsley

Large casserole dish with lid • Large saucepan • Sieve, potato ricer or masher

Prepare and cook the base • Peel and dice the onions and garlic • Cut the carrots into chunks • Heat the olive oil in a large casserole dish over a medium heat • Add the onions, garlic, carrots and a pinch of salt • Mix well and cook for about 10 minutes until the carrots begin to turn soft

Prepare and cook the meat and mushrooms • Cut the plant-based steaks into bite-sized chunks • Mix the plant-based bacon lardons and plant-based steak through the vegetables and cook for 10 minutes • Cut the mushrooms in half and add to the pan along with the drained pearl onions • Mix well and cook for another 8 minutes before adding the tomato purée

Finish the boeuf bourguignon • Mix the vegetable stock pot with the boiling water and stir until completely dissolved • Pour the red wine and the stock into the casserole dish, add the thyme or rosemary sprigs, bay leaves, tamari and brown sugar and mix through • Bring the mixture to the boil, then reduce the temperature and simmer for 30 minutes, and preheat oven to 100°C • Cover and place in the oven for 30 minutes, or until ready to serve

Make the mashed potato • Peel and cut the potatoes into bite-sized pieces • Add to a large saucepan of salted boiling water over a medium heat and cook for 15 minutes, or until the potatoes are completely soft • Drain the potatoes and place into a sieve over the empty pan • Using the back of a spoon, push the potatoes through the sieve and collect in the pan below (alternatively, use a potato ricer or masher) • Scrape any potato off the base of the sieve • Add the butter and mix through until melted • Add the milk and mix through until well combined • Taste and season with salt and pepper, adding a dash more milk if needed, until you reach your favourite consistency

Time to serve • Remove the thyme or rosemary sprigs and bay leaves from the boeuf bourguignon • Spoon the boeuf bourguignon into serving bowls and add a side of creamy mashed potato • Chop the parsley, if using, and sprinkle over the top with some black pepper

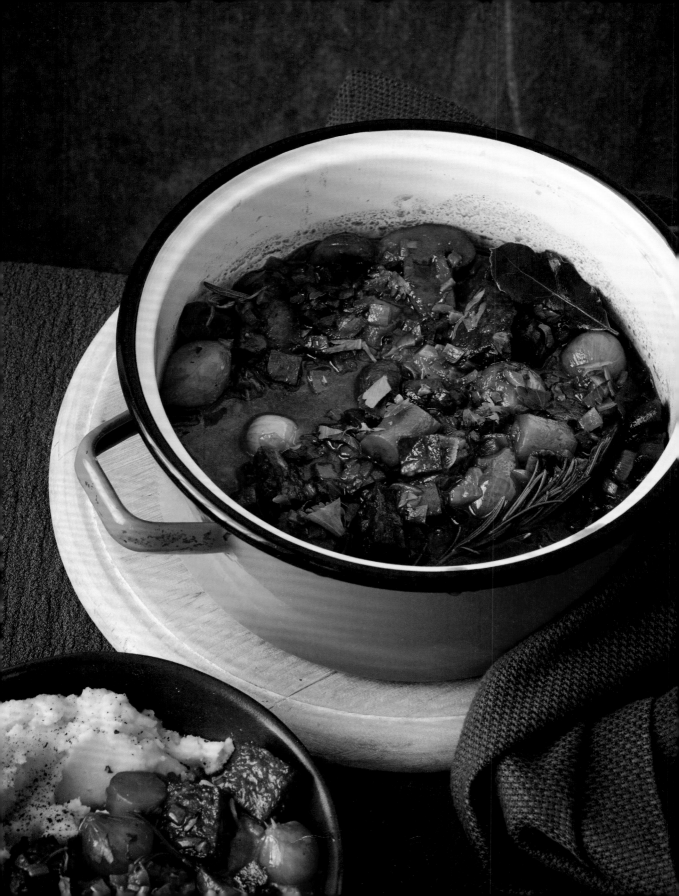

SOUTH AFRICAN BOBOTIE

Bobotie is a traditional South African dish that's kinda like a lasagne and kinda like a moussaka but actually not really like either. The dish is made with curried mince and lentils spiced with ginger, turmeric, cinnamon and mango chutney topped with a set savoury custard layer – it's the most epic sharing dish. We serve it with bright yellow rice, flavoured with turmeric and lemon, for the perfect meal. It's got a really nice fragrance, a gorgeous colour and beautiful texture. If you're a creative cook who's craving a little tasty challenge, give this a whirl. We think bobotie is brilliant and we hope you do too!

SERVES 4–6

FOR THE TOPPING
2 x 300g packs silken tofu
2 tbsp nooch (nutritional yeast)
½ tsp ground turmeric
sea salt

FOR THE BASE
2 onions
3 garlic cloves
splash of olive oil
2 carrots
1 heaped tbsp mild curry powder
½ tsp ground turmeric
½ tsp ground ginger
½ tsp ground cinnamon
1 tsp ground coriander
1 tsp hot chilli powder (optional, for a kick of spice)
½ tsp dried mixed herbs
1 x 400g tin green lentils
600g plant-based mince
1 tbsp apple cider vinegar
4 tbsp mango chutney
4 bay leaves
sea salt and black pepper

FOR THE RICE
140g jasmine rice
25g plant-based butter
1 tbsp olive oil
280ml water
1 tsp ground turmeric
1 tsp caster sugar
1 lemon
100g golden raisins
sea salt

Powerful food processor • Large saucepan with lid • Large ovenproof dish • Medium saucepan with lid • Box grater and fine grater or microplane

Make the topping • Drain the silken tofu and place it into a powerful food processor • Add the nooch, a pinch of salt and the turmeric • Blend the mixture until really smooth • Leave to one side until needed

Make the base • Peel and finely dice the onions and garlic • Place a large saucepan over a medium heat and add the olive oil • Add the diced onion, garlic and a pinch of salt • Mix well and cook for 5–10 minutes until the onion begins to soften • Grate in the carrots and cook for 5 minutes before mixing through the spices and mixed herbs and cooking for another few minutes • Preheat oven to 180°C • Drain the lentils and add them to the pan with the plant-based mince then mix well, breaking up the mince with a wooden spoon • Mix well until everything is well combined and cook for 10–15 minutes until the plant-based mince has browned • Add the apple cider vinegar, mango chutney and 2 of the bay leaves • Taste and season with salt and lots of pepper

Assemble the bobotie • Spoon the base mixture into a large ovenproof dish then top with the silken tofu topping • Smooth over the top with a large spoon and place the remaining 2 bay leaves on top

Cook the bobotie • Place the bobotie on the top shelf of the oven and cook for 15–20 minutes, or until the top turns golden brown

Cook the rice • Rinse the rice in a sieve under cold running water for 1 minute • Place a medium saucepan over a medium heat and add the butter • Once melted, add the tablespoon of olive oil and the rice, mix well and toast for a couple of seconds before pouring in the water and adding the turmeric and sugar • Bring the rice and the water to the boil • Once boiling, reduce the heat to a low simmer and cover the pan with a lid • Cook for 12 minutes, or until all of the water has been absorbed by the rice • After 12 minutes, remove from the heat and leave the rice to rest for 10 minutes with the lid on

Time to serve • Fluff the rice with a fork • Grate in some of the lemon zest then halve the lemon and add a squeeze of lemon juice, catching any pips with your free hand • Add the raisins and season with some salt • Spoon the rice into a large serving bowl and serve alongside the bobotie

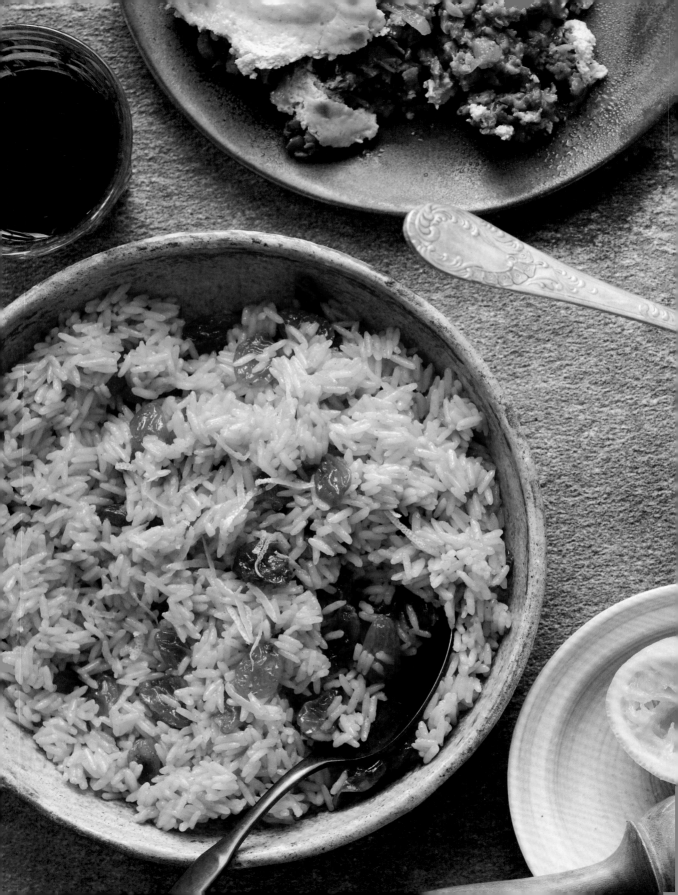

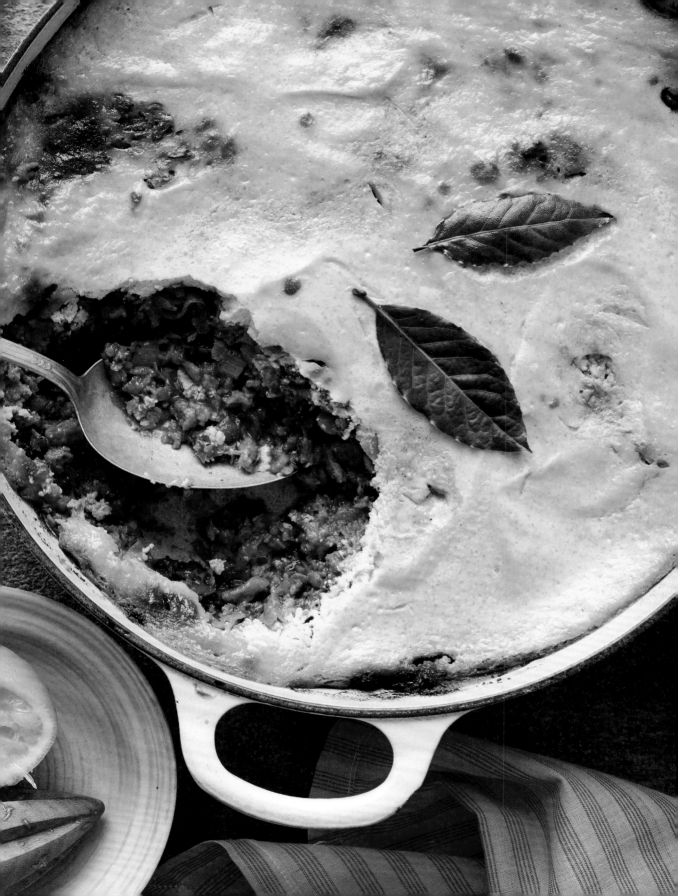

BBQ SMASH BURGERS

Ian's dad Neil used to make rissoles for tea every now and again and they were delicious. These BBQ Smash Burgers are loosely based on Neil's rissoles but we've tweaked them a little by lacing them with BBQ sauce for a smoky-sweet twist. These burgers will put a smile on your face over and over again. Brioche buns stacked high with homemade patties, sliced tomato, BBQ mayo, crispy fried onions, chopped lettuce and melted plant-based cheese for the ultimate burger experience.

MAKES 4 MEGA BURGERS OR 8 REGULAR BURGERS

FOR THE PATTIES
4 echalion shallots
2 tbsp olive oil, plus extra
    for greasing your hands
1 tbsp brown sugar
600g plant-based mince
50g breadcrumbs
50g BBQ sauce
sea salt and black pepper

FOR THE BURGERS
4–8 plant-based brioche
    buns
4 tbsp olive oil
1 romaine lettuce
1 beef tomato (or large
    tomato)
4 tbsp plant-based
    mayonnaise
4 tbsp BBQ sauce
4–8 plant-based cheese
    slices
crispy fried onions

Preheat oven to 180°C • Frying pan • Baking tray lined with baking parchment • Wide, flat-bottomed glass

Make the patties • Peel and finely dice the shallots • Place a frying pan over a medium heat and add the olive oil • Once warm, add the shallots and a pinch of salt • Mix well and cook for 3–4 minutes until soft • Add the brown sugar to the pan and cook for a further 3–4 minutes until the shallots have caramelised • Once cooked, take the pan off the heat, spoon the shallots into a bowl and leave to cool for a few minutes • To the bowl, add the plant-based mince, breadcrumbs, BBQ sauce and season with salt and pepper • Mix until well combined

Shape the patties • Lightly oil your hands and shape the mixture into 4 plump patties or 8 smaller patties • Set the patties out on a lined baking tray and 'smash' them with the base of a wide, flat-bottomed glass – if needed you can shape the sides neatly using your hands • Cook in the oven for 25 minutes

Prepare the remaining ingredients • Halve the brioche buns • Drizzle the cut sides with the olive oil and toast in the frying pan over a high heat until golden brown • Remove the core of the lettuce and shred the leaves • Thinly slice the tomato • In a small bowl, mix together the plant-based mayo and BBQ sauce until smooth

Finish the burgers • After 25 minutes, remove the tray from the oven • Place the plant-based cheese slices on top of the burger patties and return the tray to the oven for 1 minute to melt the cheese

Time to serve • Cover one half of the burger buns with the BBQ mayo • Take the patties out of the oven and transfer to the burger buns • Dress the burgers with sliced lettuce, tomato and crispy fried onions • Close the burgers and serve immediately

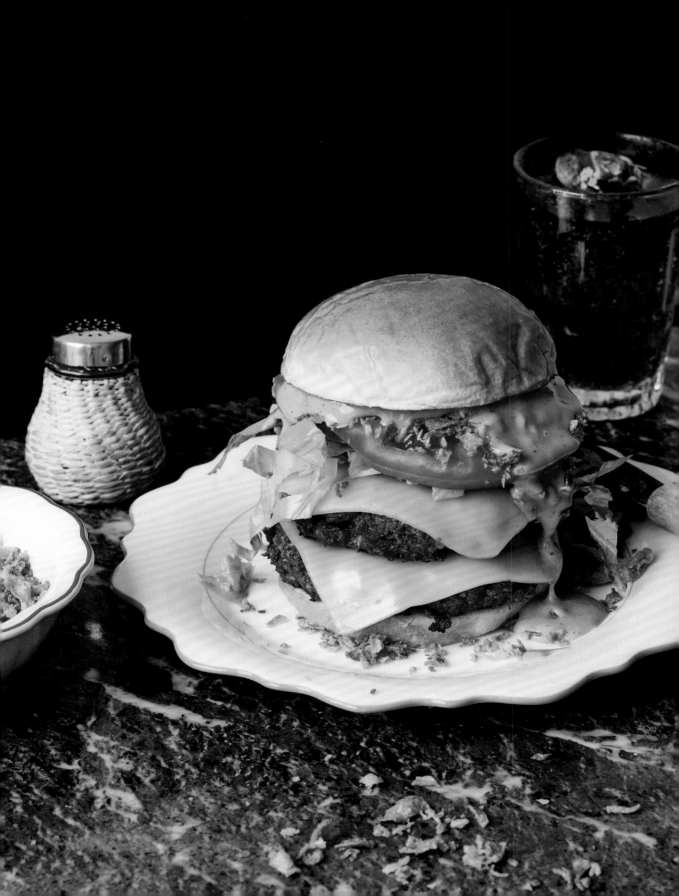

CRISPY SHREDDED BEEF WITH EGG-FRIED RICE

This is quite simply one of the best fakeaways we've done. It might be worth buying some takeaway boxes so you can complete the Friday-night Chinese takeaway experience. The sweet, sticky sauce on the crispy beef strips creates one of the most moreish bites you'll ever try. We serve it with egg-fried rice, made from crumbling tofu with turmeric-infused rice, with some vegetables for an added touch of freshness. Kick your shoes off, whack the telly on and dig into this downright delicious dish; you deserve it.

SERVES 4

FOR THE MARINADE
2 tbsp tamari
2 tsp shop-bought ginger
    and garlic paste
2 tbsp toasted sesame oil
½ tsp caster sugar

FOR THE BEEF
400g plant-based beef
140g cornflour
200ml vegetable oil
    (for frying)
sea salt

FOR THE RICE
150g jasmine rice
25g plant-based butter
1 tbsp olive oil
300ml cold water
1 tsp light brown sugar
1 onion
2 garlic cloves
1 red pepper
drizzle of toasted sesame oil
½ block of firm tofu (140g)
1 tsp ground turmeric
2 tsp tamari
100g frozen peas
sea salt

**FOR THE STIR-FRY
SAUCE**
3 tbsp sweet chilli sauce
2 tbsp regular or
    spicy ketchup
2 tbsp tamari
1 tbsp brown sugar or
    maple syrup
1 tbsp rice vinegar
1 tsp sea salt

TO SERVE
1 red chilli
handful of coriander
4 spring onions

Large saucepan • 3 large frying pans • Slotted spoon

Marinate the beef and prep the vegetables • Mix all the marinade ingredients in a large bowl • If using beef 'steak', cut it into strips max 1cm thick • Add the plant-based meat to the marinade, mix well and set aside for 10–15 minutes

Cook the rice • Rinse the rice in a sieve under cold running water for 1 minute • Place a large saucepan over a medium heat and add the butter • Add the olive oil and the rice, mix well and toast for a couple of seconds before pouring in the water and adding the sugar • Cover, bring to the boil then turn the heat down to a low simmer and cook for 12 minutes, or until all of the water is absorbed • After 12 minutes, leave the rice to rest for 10 minutes with the lid on • Place to one side until needed (see note on cooking rice below)

Make the stir-fry sauce • Combine all the ingredients in a bowl until lump free

Coat the beef • One by one, remove the plant-based meat strips from the marinade, drip dry for a second (if necessary) then place in a large bowl or baking tray • Coat all over with the cornflour • Reserve the leftover marinade

Fry the rice • Peel and dice the onion and garlic, deseed and cut the pepper into small cubes • Heat the sesame oil in a large frying pan over a medium heat • Add the diced onion, garlic, pepper cubes and a pinch of salt • Mix well and cook for 5–10 minutes until the onion softens • Crumble in the tofu, add the turmeric and mix through • Cook for a few minutes then mix through the cooked rice, tamari and peas • Cook for 5–10 minutes until piping hot

Cook the beef • Heat the 200ml vegetable oil in a separate large frying pan over a high heat then add the marinated meat strips • Shallow-fry the strips for 2–4 minutes until very crispy, turning them frequently • Once cooked, remove the strips from the oil with a slotted spoon and transfer to kitchen paper

Coat the beef • Place another saucepan over a high heat • Add the stir-fry sauce and remaining marinade and cook for a couple of minutes until thick and sticky • Add the beef strips and mix well to coat

Time to serve • Thinly slice the chilli and coriander and trim and thinly slice the spring onions • Spoon the fried rice in dishes and serve with the crispy beef • Sprinkle sliced red chilli, coriander and spring onions over the top

NOTE
Don't leave cooked rice out at room temperature for long. If necessary, place the rice in the fridge and reheat to a very hot temperature when ready to serve.

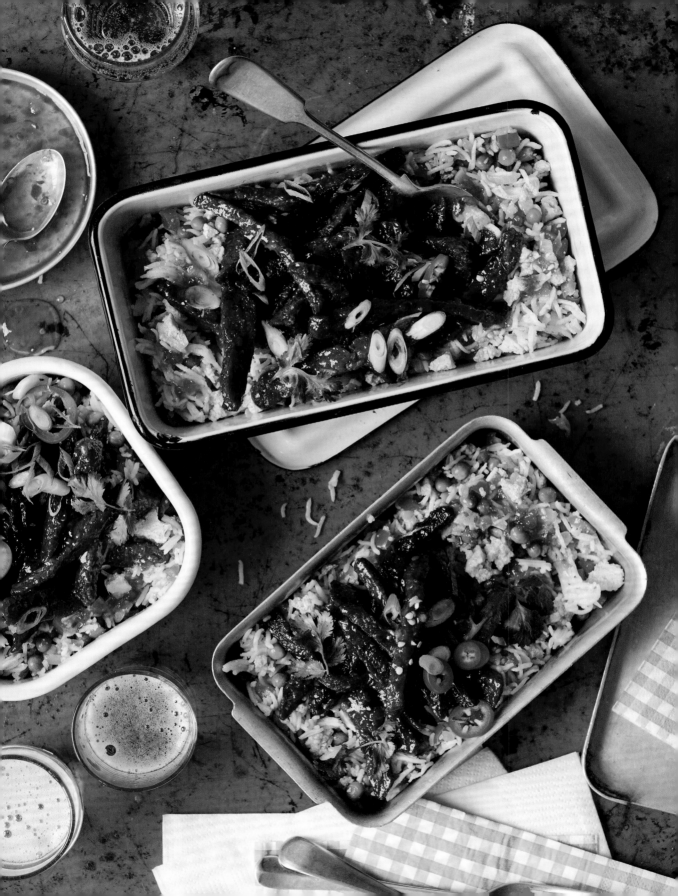

BIG BOSH MEATY SUNDAY LUNCH

There's nothing better than getting your nearest and dearest around a table to share a good meal on a Sunday afternoon. It's the perfect place to tell stories, discuss ideas and just catch up. This is the meatiest plant-based wellington you will ever try, with a mince-based filling encased in a layer of mushrooms and crispy golden pastry. It's served with the ultimate sides – creamy and cheesy leeks, maple-roasted parsnips, moreish bacon sprouts and THE perfect crispy roast potatoes, topped with a rich red onion gravy to bring everything together. If you haven't hosted a Sunday lunch for a while, why don't you call a few friends or family, arrange a date, invite them over and cook them this? We guarantee you won't regret it.

You can get ahead and prep the wellington the day before you want to serve it.

If you're making the wellington to serve 8, scale up the sides by 20%.

WELLINGTON

SERVES 6-8

FOR THE FILLING
900g meaty plant-based
   burgers (about 4 packs)
2 tbsp olive oil
sea salt and black pepper
Dijon mustard, for brushing
   the beef

FOR THE MUSHROOM DUXELLES
650g chestnut mushrooms
180g cooked chestnuts
1 garlic clove, peeled
drizzle of olive oil
2 thyme sprigs
sea salt and black pepper

TO ASSEMBLE
2 x ready-rolled plant-based
   puff pastry sheets
unsweetened almond milk,
   for brushing
mixed black and white
   sesame seeds

Baking tray • Food processor • Large frying pan • Large baking sheet • Pastry brush

Make the wellington • Put the plant-based burger patties in a large mixing bowl • Season with salt and pepper and mash with a fork until they all break down and come together • Use your hands to shape them into one thick sausage shape that will make up the 'fillet' in the wellington • Wrap the sausage in cling film, place on a baking tray and put into the fridge to firm up while you make the mushroom duxelles

Make the mushroom duxelles • Clean and halve the chestnut mushrooms, then add them to a food processor with the cooked chestnuts, garlic clove and a pinch each of salt and pepper and blend to a paste • Heat the drizzle of oil in a large frying pan over a high heat • Once warm, add the mushroom paste, pick the leaves from the thyme sprigs and add them too • Mix well and cook for 5–10 minutes, stirring every now and then, until the paste has dried out • Once cooked, leave to one side to cool

While the mushroom duxelles is cooling, seal the fillet • Wipe out the pan you made the duxelles in and heat a drizzle of olive oil in the pan over a high heat • Remove the cling film from the fillet and add it to the pan • Sear on each side until evenly browned all over • Transfer to a plate and brush all over with Dijon mustard, then set aside

Make the wellington filling • Lay a large piece of cling film on your work surface and spread the mushroom mixture on top to the width of the fillet • Lay the fillet at the edge of the mushroom layer • Tightly roll the fillet into a sausage shape • Twist the ends of the cling film so it holds tightly together, then refrigerate for 15 minutes to firm up

Finish the wellington • Unroll one sheet of puff pastry onto a large baking sheet, keeping the paper on the bottom • Unwrap the fillet from the cling film and place it on the middle of the pastry sheet • Brush almond milk a thumbs-width around the edge of the fillet

Place another pastry sheet over the top of the fillet and press down around the base where the almond milk has been brushed to seal the two pastry sheets together • Cut around the edge of the pastry, a thumbs-width from the fillet, to make a neat border, keeping any leftover pastry to decorate • Wrap the wellington tightly in cling film and chill for another 10 minutes, or overnight if you're super organised • Preheat oven to 190°C

Glaze the wellington • Remove the cling film and decorate the pastry with the off-cuts if you like, re-rolling and cutting them as necessary – we like to cover the wellington in pastry strips placed diagonally across the top • Make a hole in the pastry with a chopstick to prevent the pastry from splitting • Glaze the wellington all over with almond milk and sprinkle with sesame seeds

Cook the wellington • Cook the wellington in the oven for 45–50 minutes, until golden and delicious

Time to serve • Rest for 15 minutes to allow the juices to settle, then transfer to a cutting board and slice

ROAST POTATOES

SERVES 6

100ml olive oil
2kg Maris Piper potatoes
2 tbsp gram flour
2 rosemary sprigs
sea salt

Preheat oven to 190°C • Large baking tray • Peeler • Large saucepan

Pour the olive oil onto a large baking tray • Place in the oven while you prepare the potatoes

Peel the potatoes and cut into big chunks • Put the potato chunks in a large saucepan over a medium heat, cover with water and add a sprinkle of salt • Bring to the boil • Once boiling, reduce the heat and cook for 2 minutes • After 2 minutes, drain the water and leave the potatoes to steam for a couple of minutes until completely dry • Once the potatoes are dry, remove the baking tray from the oven and add the drained potatoes (being really careful because the oil will be hot) and mix to coat • Roast the potatoes for 25 minutes • After 25 minutes, mix through the gram flour, a good pinch of sea salt and the rosemary sprigs • Mix well and roast for another 20–30 minutes, until golden, crispy and delicious

MAPLE-ROASTED PARSNIPS AND CARROTS

SERVES 6

3 large carrots
3 large parsnips
drizzle of olive oil
40g ground almonds
2 tbsp maple syrup
50g toasted pine nuts
10g flat-leaf parsley
sea salt and black pepper

Preheat oven to 190°C • Large baking tray

Cut the carrots and parsnips into bite-sized chunks • Put the chunks on a large baking tray and add the drizzle of olive oil and a pinch of salt • Mix well until all of the ingredients are coated in the olive oil and cook in the oven for 35 minutes • After 35 minutes, mix through the ground almonds and maple syrup, and return to the oven for another 5–10 minutes until golden and cooked through • Remove from the oven and mix through the pine nuts (saving some for the top) • Chop the parsley • Spoon onto a serving plate and sprinkle with the chopped parsley and some black pepper

GRAVY

SERVES 6

1 plant-based beef stock
    pot or OXO cube
300ml boiling water, plus
    extra when needed
3 red onions
4 garlic cloves
drizzle of olive oil
2 tsp steak seasoning
1 vegetable stock pot
3 tbsp tomato purée
400ml plant-based red wine
    (mild flavoured)
3 rosemary sprigs
2 large bay leaves (or 3 small)
1 tbsp yeast extract
    (we use Marmite)
2 tsp light brown sugar
sea salt

Large saucepan • Sieve (optional)

Mix the beef stock pot with the boiling water until completely dissolved • Peel and finely dice the onions, peel and dice the garlic • Place a large saucepan over a medium heat and add the olive oil • Once warm, add the onions, garlic and a pinch of salt • Mix well and cook for 5–10 minutes until the onions start to soften • Add the steak seasoning, vegetable stock pot, tomato purée, red wine, beef stock, rosemary, bay leaves, yeast extract and brown sugar • Bring to the boil then reduce the heat and simmer for 20 minutes, adding a splash of water whenever the gravy becomes too thick (we add about 200ml) • Pass the gravy through a sieve (optional, for a smooth gravy) • Once ready to serve, heat the gravy over a medium heat and top up with water until it reaches the consistency you like best (we add about 150ml water)

BACON SPROUTS

SERVES 6

600g Brussels sprouts
1 x 150g pack
    plant-based bacon
drizzle of olive oil
small knob of
    plant-based butter
½ tbsp maple syrup
½ lemon
grated plant-based
    parmesan (optional)
sea salt and black pepper

Preheat oven to 190°C • Large baking dish • Medium saucepan

Halve the sprouts and cut the bacon into chunks • Place the sprouts into a large baking dish, drizzle with the olive oil and sprinkle with a good pinch of salt • Mix well until all of the sprouts are coated • Roast in the oven for 15–25 minutes, or until the sprouts are golden and crispy on the outside and cooked through • While the sprouts are roasting, place a medium saucepan over a medium heat and add the butter • Once melted, add the bacon chunks, mix well and cook for 5 minutes (or however long it states on the packet) • Once the sprouts are cooked, remove them from the oven and mix through the pan of bacon • Add the maple syrup and a squeeze of lemon juice (catching any pips in your free hand) and mix again until everything comes together • Spoon the sprouts onto a serving plate and top with some grated plant-based parmesan (if using) and a pinch of black pepper

CREAMY LEEKS

SERVES 6

3 leeks
small knob of
    plant-based butter
100g frozen peas
100g plant-based crème
    fraîche (or cream)
3 tbsp nooch (nutritional
    yeast) or plant-based
    parmesan
2 tsp Dijon mustard
½ lemon
sea salt

Medium saucepan

Trim and thinly slice the leeks • Place a medium saucepan over a medium heat and add the butter • Once melted, add the sliced leeks and a pinch of salt • Mix well and cook for 5–10 minutes, or until the leeks soften • Once soft, mix through the frozen peas, plant-based crème fraîche (or cream), nooch (or parmesan), mustard and a squeeze of lemon juice (catching any pips in your free hand) • Reduce the heat and cook for a few more minutes, or until everything comes together and the peas soften • Taste and season accordingly • Once cooked, spoon into a dish and serve hot

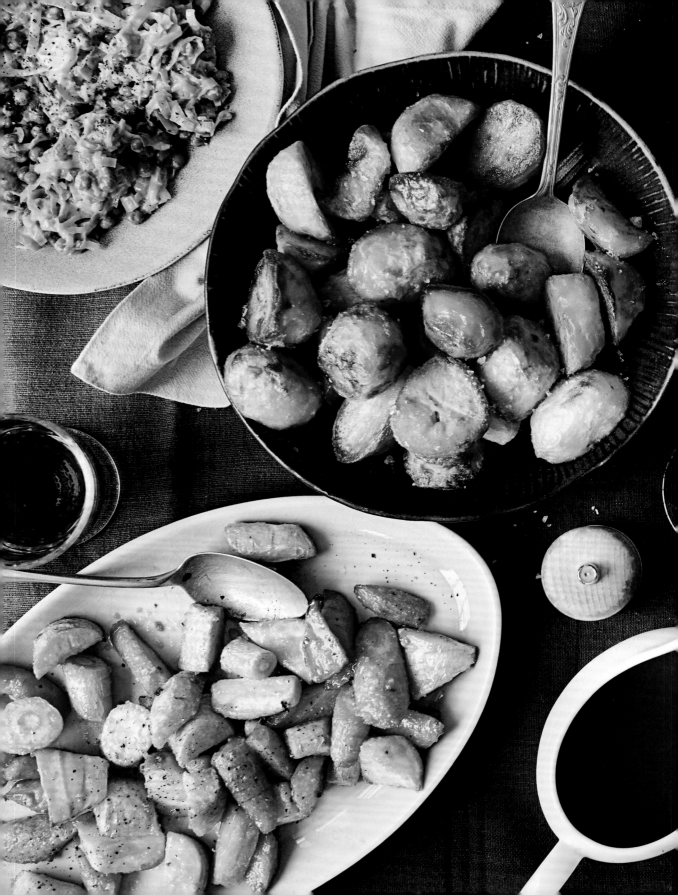

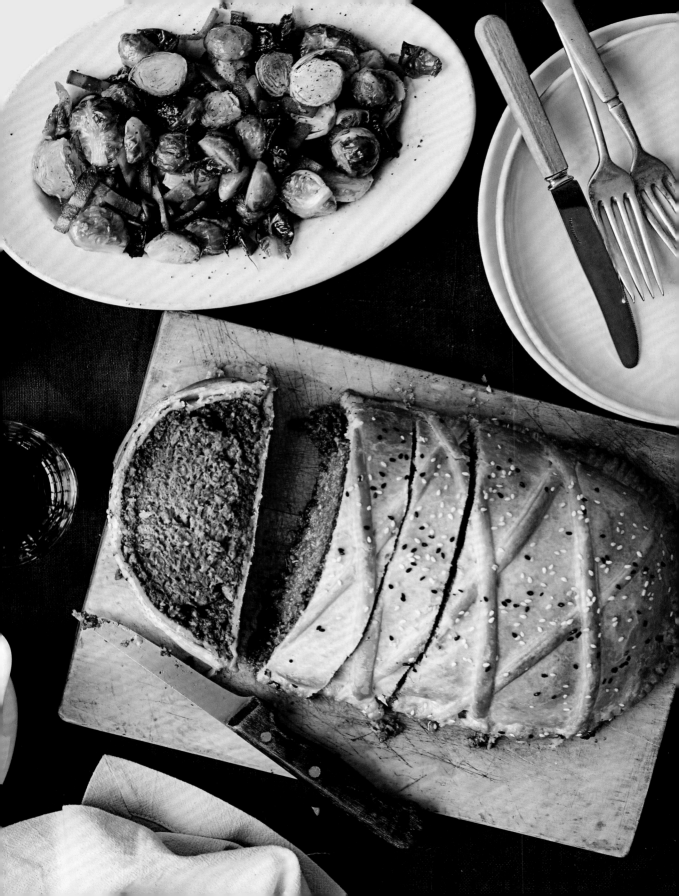

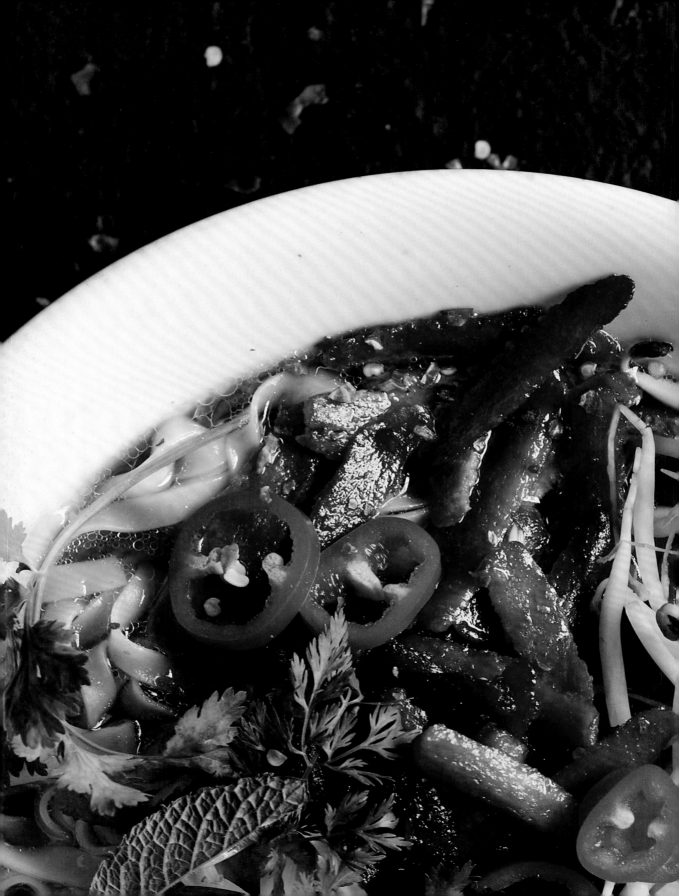

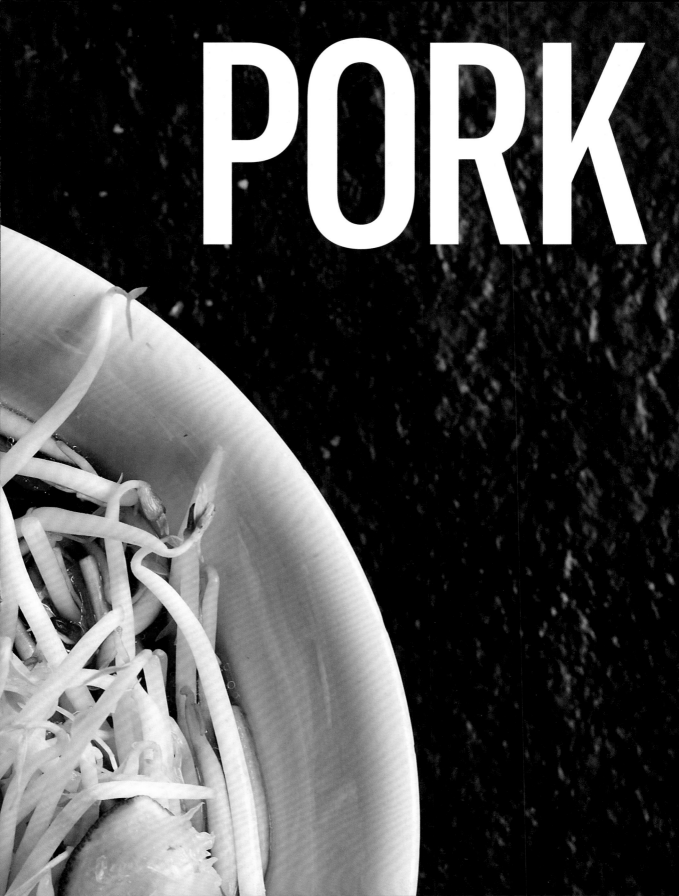

PORK

PILLOWY PORK STEAMED BUNS

These little beauties are super fun to make and a real joy to eat. The filling is zippy and sweet, and the buns are soft and squidgy. Rip 'em, dip 'em and chow down for ultimate smile-inducing satisfaction.

SERVES 4 (MAKES 8 BUNS)

FOR THE DOUGH
300g plain flour, plus extra for dusting
1 tsp fast-action dried yeast
1 tsp caster sugar
160–180g warm water
200ml water in a separate small bowl (optional)

FOR THE FILLING
2½ tbsp light soy sauce, plus extra to serve
1 tbsp Shaoxing wine
2½ tbsp hoisin sauce
1–2 tsp caster sugar, to taste
¼ tsp Chinese five-spice
generous pinch of ground black pepper
1 tbsp rice wine vinegar
3 small shallots
2 garlic cloves
thumb-sized piece of ginger
1 tbsp vegetable oil
200g plant-based mince (ideally pork)
1 tsp toasted sesame oil
salt
white sesame seeds, for sprinkling (optional)

Microwave • Fine grater or microplane • Large heavy-based frying pan or wok • Rolling pin • Large saucepan • Bamboo steamer • Baking parchment • Kettle boiled

Prepare the dough • Put the flour in a mixing bowl and set to one side • Add the yeast, sugar and warm water to a jug, stir to combine and leave to activate for 1 minute • Add the liquid to the bowl of flour and stir with a wooden spoon until the mixture comes together to form a smooth dough • Tip the dough out onto the kitchen surface and knead for 10 minutes until smooth and supple • Place the dough back in the bowl and cover with cling film • Leave to rise in a warm place for 1 hour or until doubled in size • If you want to speed up the proving process, place the second bowl of water in the microwave and heat on full power for 1½ minutes • Remove the bowl from the microwave, place the bowl of dough in the microwave (still covered with cling film), shut the door and leave to prove for 30 minutes

Prepare the filling • Mix the soy sauce, Shaoxing wine, hoisin sauce, sugar, Chinese five-spice, pepper and vinegar in a bowl • Peel and finely dice the shallots • Peel and grate the garlic and ginger • Warm the vegetable oil in a frying pan or wok over a medium heat, add the shallots and stir for 1 minute • Add the garlic and ginger and stir-fry for a minute until the mix becomes aromatic • Add the pork mince and the toasted sesame oil and stir for a couple of minutes, breaking up the mince using a wooden spoon • Reduce the heat, add the sauce, stir everything together and cook for 3–5 minutes, then season and set aside to cool

Form the buns • Divide the dough into 8 equal pieces, roll each into a ball and place a damp tea towel over the balls to stop them drying out • Take a piece of dough and press it into a 12cm disc (quite like a small pizza base) sprinkle over a little flour and use a rolling pin to roll out the edges, turning them 20 degrees with each roll – this method should give you a small disc that's a little thicker in the middle • Place an eighth of the filling into the middle of the disc and crimp the edges around the top of the filling to form a plump, pillowy bun

Cook the buns and serve • Cut baking parchment into steamer-shaped circles then cut holes in the circles to allow steam to penetrate • Drizzle a little oil over the paper circles and place in a bamboo steamer • Add a 5cm depth of boiling water to a large saucepan and keep it bubbling over a high heat • Top the pan with the bamboo steamer, place the buns in the steamer (steam them in batches if necessary), put the lid on and steam for 11–12 minutes • Take the bamboo steamer off the heat and leave the steamed buns to rest for 2 minutes before serving with extra soy sauce for dipping, scattered with sesame seeds if you like

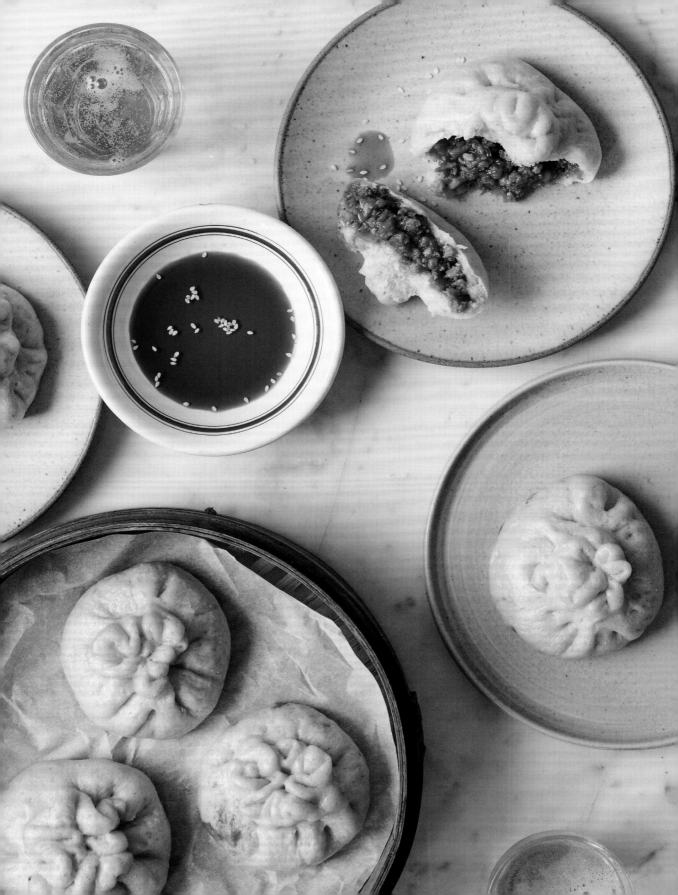

CHORIZO BANGERS WITH BUTTERBEAN MASH

Spanish-style bangers and mash that everyone will love. Good bangers deserve great accompaniments and with this recipe that's exactly what you get. Thick, aromatic gravy spiced with saffron and harissa, served with creamy, paprika mash and a lovely selection of lemony red peppers and olives – we guarantee every bite will be different from the next.

SERVES 4

1 x 216g pack plant-based
   chorizo sausages

FOR THE GRAVY
pinch of saffron threads
2 veggie stock cubes
500ml boiling water, plus
   a splash more when
   needed
4 red onions
3 garlic cloves
drizzle of olive oil
pinch of sea salt
1 tsp paprika
½–1 tsp light brown sugar
2 tsp rose harissa paste
1 tbsp tomato purée
1 tbsp red wine vinegar
sea salt

FOR THE MASH
1 onion
2 garlic cloves
drizzle of olive oil
2 x 400g tins butterbeans
2 tsp smoked paprika
50g plant-based butter
175ml plant-based cream,
   plus extra if needed
2 tbsp nooch (nutritional
   yeast)
1 tsp rose harissa paste
1 lemon
sea salt

FOR THE PEPPERS
1 red pepper
1 yellow pepper
handful of pitted
   black olives
drizzle of olive oil
½ lemon
sea salt (optional)

FOR THE TOP
handful of parsley
black pepper

2 large frying pans • Hand blender, potato masher or blender

Make the gravy • Mix the saffron and stock cubes with the boiling water until dissolved • Peel and finely dice 2 of the onions, peel and slice the remaining 2 • Peel and dice the garlic • Place a large frying pan over a medium heat and add the drizzle of olive oil • Once warm, add all of the onions, the garlic and a pinch of salt • Mix well and cook for about 10 minutes, or until the onions soften • Mix through the paprika and cook for another couple of seconds before pouring in the stock and adding the sugar, harissa paste, tomato purée and red wine vinegar • Reduce the heat and simmer the gravy for at least 30 minutes, adding a dash of water if the mixture ever feels like it's becoming too thick

Make the mash • Peel and slice the onion, peel and dice the garlic • Place a large frying pan over a medium heat and add the olive oil • Once warm, add the sliced onion, garlic and a pinch of salt, mix well and cook for 10 minutes until the onion begins to soften • Drain the butterbeans and add to the pan along with the paprika • Mix well and cook for 10 minutes, or until the butterbeans begin to break down • At this point, add the butter, plant-based cream, nooch and harissa paste • Halve the lemon and squeeze in the juice of both halves, catching any pips in your free hand • Use a hand blender or potato masher (or spoon the mixture into a blender) and blend until the mixture comes together to create a really smooth mash

Cook the peppers • Halve, core and thinly slice the peppers and halve the olives • Place a large frying pan over a medium heat (you can transfer the gravy to a jug and use the pan for the peppers) and add the olive oil • Add the sliced peppers and olives and cook for 10 minutes, or until they begin to soften • Squeeze in some lemon juice, catching any pips in your free hand, and season if needed

Cook the sausages • Cook the sausages according to the instructions on the packet

Time to serve • Divide the mash among plates and top with the sausages • Spoon on the red peppers and top the whole thing with a good amount of gravy • Chop the parsley and sprinkle on top, as well as some black pepper

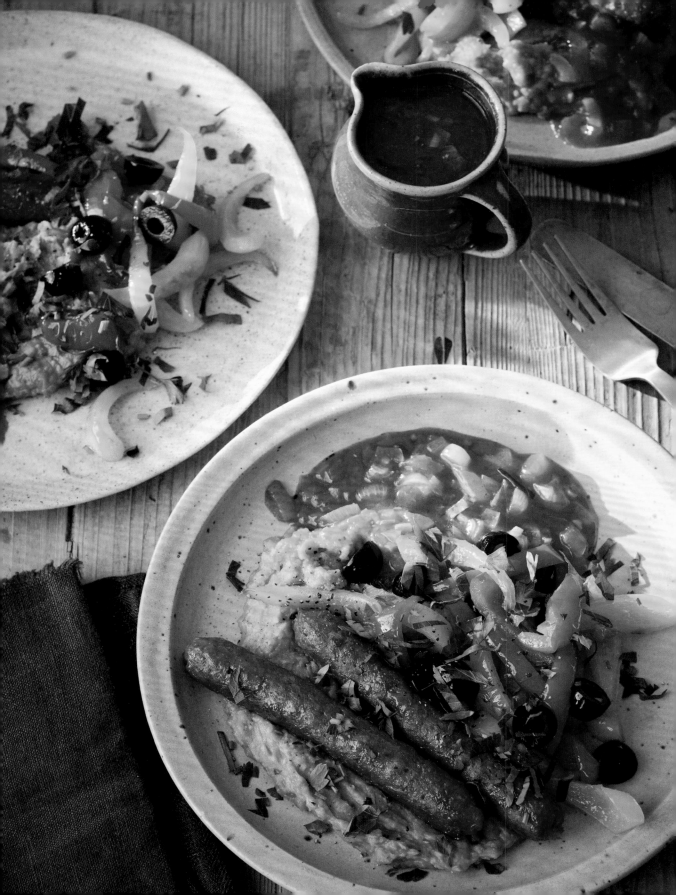

PHO KING

Soupy noodles are such a treat, we eat them all the time! Loaded with deliciousness and bursting with goodness, they're marvellously slurpable, sensationally satisfying and surprisingly straightforward to make. The broth is where the love goes into this dish, made by simmering down fresh ginger, cinnamon sticks, star anise, cloves and miso paste to make the perfect pho base that fills your kitchen with the most exquisite smells. Come to think of it, these little beauties might be the best Pho King noodles you've ever tasted.

SERVES 2

FOR THE BROTH
knob of fresh ginger
2 cinnamon sticks
2 star anise
2 cloves
1 onion
3 garlic cloves
splash of toasted sesame oil
   (or a plain-flavoured oil
   like rapeseed)
2 tbsp brown sugar
2 tbsp brown rice miso
   paste
4 tbsp tamari
2 vegetable stock pots
1 litre boiling water
1 lime
sea salt

FOR THE PHO
1 x 200g pack plant-based
   pork pieces (or beef
   pieces)
2 tbsp toasted sesame oil
1 tbsp tamari
1 tbsp light brown sugar
150g thick or thin rice
   noodles, depending on
   your preference
150g beansprouts

TO SERVE
1 red chilli
1 lime
bunch of fresh coriander
bunch of fresh mint
sriracha or a pinch of
   dried chilli flakes

Stock pan • Large saucepan • Small saucepan for noodles • Sieve

Make the broth • Peel the ginger and add to a stock pan over a medium heat, along with the cinnamon sticks, star anise and cloves • Toast the spices for about 5 minutes, until aromatic • Transfer the spices to a bowl until needed • Peel and dice the onion and garlic • Place the pan back over a low-medium heat and add the oil • Add the onion, garlic and a pinch of salt • Mix well and cook for 5–10 minutes until the onion begins to soften and become translucent • Add the brown sugar, miso paste, tamari, vegetable stock pots and boiling water • Halve the lime and squeeze in the juice • Mix well until everything comes together and the stock pots have completely dissolved • Add the ginger, cinnamon sticks, star anise and cloves back to the pan • Bring to the boil then reduce the temperature and cook at a very low simmer for 30 minutes

Cook the pork • Cut the pork into thin slices • In a small bowl, combine the sesame oil with the tamari until smooth • Add the pork and mix well until all of the pork is coated in the sauce • Place a large saucepan over a medium heat • Once the pan feels hot, add the pork slices and cook according to the timings on the packet • Add the brown sugar, mix well and leave to caramelise for a few minutes

Cook the noodles • Cook the noodles according to the instructions on the packet

Time to serve • If needed, add about a cup of water to the broth to balance the flavour • Thinly slice the red chilli and cut the lime into wedges • Pull some leaves off the coriander and mint • Strain the hot stock through a sieve • Divide the pork, beansprouts and noodles between 2 deep bowls and pour in equal amounts of the broth • Top each with a handful of mint, coriander, sliced chilli and a lime wedge on the side • Add a dash of sriracha sauce or a pinch of dried chilli flakes for a spicy kick

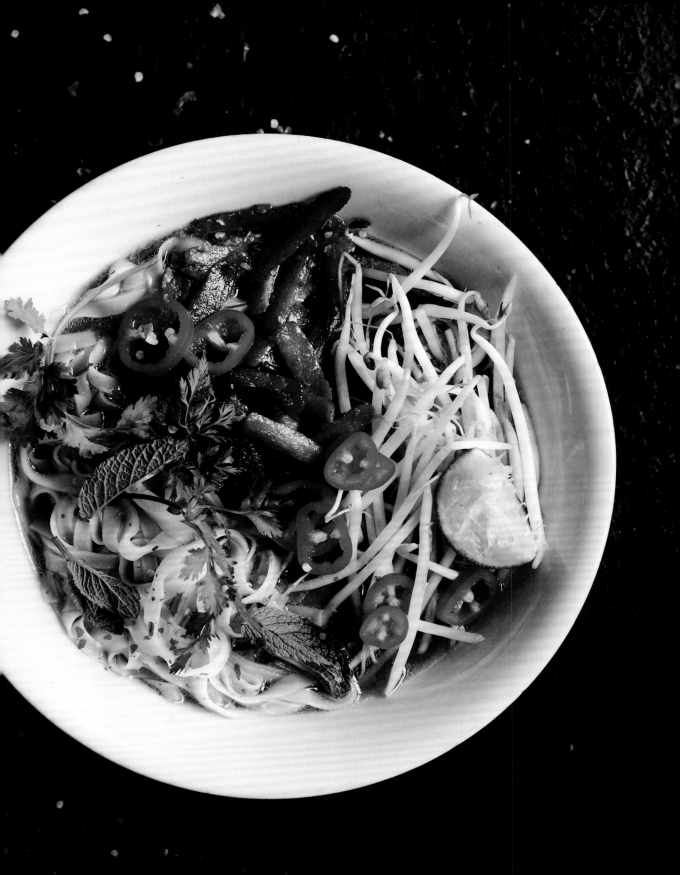

CHAR SUI PORK

This one's got a really interesting flavour profile. There's sweetness but there's also an unusual sharpness that's sure to please your palate. Perfectly cooked, simple basmati rice complements the complexity of the pork nicely, and the pak choi offers up a lovely freshness. This is a well-rounded dish that we're sure you'll love.

SERVES 4

FOR THE PORK
3 garlic cloves
55g granulated white sugar
2 tsp sea salt
½ tsp Chinese five-spice
¼ tsp ground white pepper
½ tsp toasted sesame oil
1 tbsp Shaoxing wine
1 tbsp hoisin sauce
1 tbsp light soy sauce
1½ tbsp molasses or black treacle
⅛ tsp plant-based red food colouring (optional)
1 tbsp hot water
450g plant-based pork pieces (preferably plain)

FOR THE RICE
300g basmati rice
600ml cold water
1 tsp fine sea salt

FOR THE PAK CHOI
4 medium pak choi
2 garlic cloves
2 tbsp toasted sesame oil

TO FINISH
4 spring onions
1 tbsp white sesame seeds

Fine grater or microplane • Preheat oven to 180°C • Wide, large ovenproof braising pan with lid • Large saucepan with lid • Frying pan

Prepare the pork • Peel and grate the garlic and put it in a mixing bowl • Add the sugar, salt, Chinese five-spice, pepper, sesame oil, Shaoxing wine, hoisin sauce, soy sauce, molasses or treacle, food colouring (if using) and water to the bowl and stir to combine • Add the pork to the bowl and fold to coat and combine • Add the contents of the bowl to a large ovenproof braising pan and cook for 8–10 minutes over a medium-low heat, stirring frequently

Cook the rice • Rinse the rice in a sieve under cold running water for 1 minute • Tip into a large saucepan, pour over the water and sprinkle in the salt • Cover and bring to the boil over a high heat • When the water starts to boil, turn down the heat to low and cook, covered, for 12 minutes • Take the pan off the heat, keep the lid on and leave to steam • When it's time to serve, remove the lid and fluff up the rice with a fork

Finish the pork • Place the braising pan in the oven to reduce the moisture content of the dish

Prepare the pak choi • Cut away the root ends of the pak choi and discard • Slice off the green leafy parts and roughly chop into ribbons • Slice the white part of the pak choi into 2.5cm pieces • Peel and grate the garlic • Sauté the white pak choi pieces with the sesame oil and a little salt in a frying pan for 1 minute • Add the grated garlic and sauté for a minute more • Add the ribboned pak choi leaves and a splash of water, take the pan off the heat and leave to wilt

Time to serve • Trim and thinly slice the spring onions • Spoon the rice, pak choi and char sui pork into bowls, sprinkle over the spring onions and sesame seeds and serve immediately

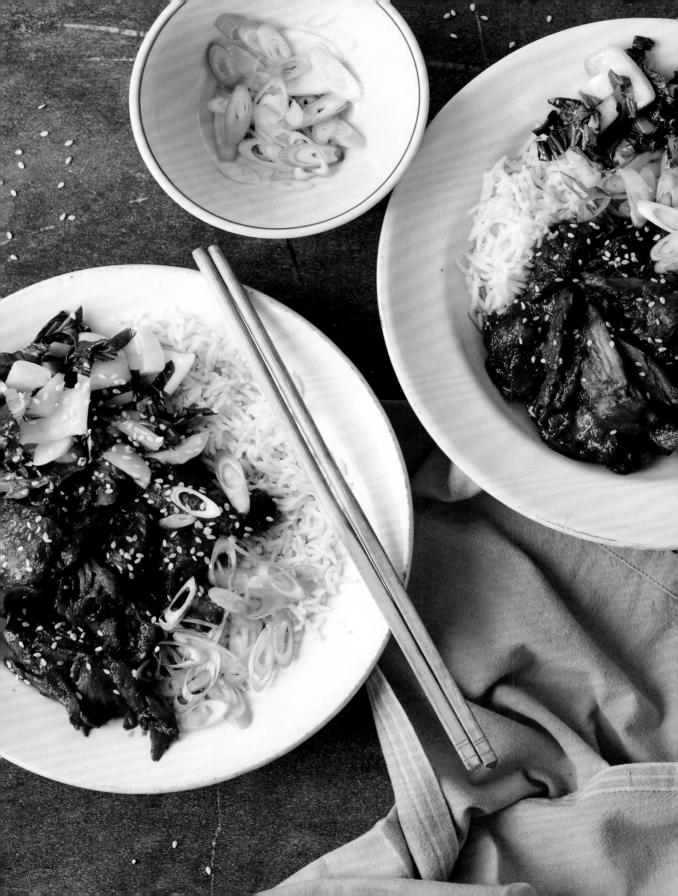

PORK BELLY AND CRACKLING WITH CARAMELISED ONION MASH AND APPLE GRAVY

If you're after a meal that requires a little work but ensures a real wow factor, this might be the one for you! It looks fabulous, it tastes fantastic and we think that if you make it, it'll end up being one of your favourites.

SERVES 2

FOR THE PORK BELLY
80g Vital wheat gluten flour
20g pea protein isolate
½ tsp sea salt
¼ tsp ground black pepper
2g garlic powder
3g smoked paprika
5g beetroot powder
110g water
6g liquid smoke
6g maple syrup
30g white miso paste

FOR THE PORK FAT
120ml coconut milk
4 tbsp tapioca starch
3 tbsp rice flour
½ tsp salt
30ml olive oil, plus
    extra for drizzling
sea salt flakes

FOR THE CRACKLING
1 sheet of tofu skin/bean
    curd sheet (10g)
1 tbsp light soy sauce
½ tsp garlic powder
½ tsp smoked paprika
¼ tsp sugar
½ tsp sea salt
¼ tsp ground black pepper
1 tbsp vegetable oil

FOR THE CARAMELISED ONION MASH
4 onions
2 garlic cloves
800g King Edward potatoes
4 tbsp vegetable oil
pinch of brown sugar (optional)
4 tbsp plant-based butter,
    plus extra to taste
90ml oat milk
sea salt and black pepper

Preheat oven to 60°C • Small metal bowl • Medium metal bowl • Rolling pin • 2 small saucepans • Medium saucepan • Steaming basket or colander • Foil • Shallow baking tray • Frying pan • Large saucepan • Hand blender, potato ricer or masher

Make the pork belly • Put a small metal bowl of water in the bottom of the oven • Whisk all the dry ingredients together in a separate medium metal bowl • Pour in the 110g water with the other wet ingredients and mix until it comes together as a rough dough, using the dough to clean the sides of the bowl of any residue • Cover the surface of the dough with cling film then wrap the bowl in cling film • Place the dough in the oven to hydrate for 1 hour – this hydration will allow you to roll out the dough without it springing back too much • Unwrap the bowl, remove the dough and roll it into a very long strip, turning it over a couple of times to help stretch the gluten • Once it's as thin as you can roll it, fold the dough back on itself at 12cm intervals so you have lots of layers • Wrap tightly in cling film

Make the pork fat • Warm the coconut milk, tapioca starch, rice flour and salt in a small saucepan over a low heat • Whisk for 3–4 minutes until you have a thick paste • Remove from the heat (it will thicken while you prepare your pork)

Cook the pork belly • Heat some water in a medium saucepan and put a steaming basket or colander on the top • Steam the pork (still wrapped in the cling film) for 1½ hours • Carefully unwrap and leave to cool for a few minutes • Heat the oven to 180°C • Once the pork has cooled, slice the meat in half and then stand each piece on its side and cut in half again to make 4 thin pieces • Assemble pieces of pork belly on 15cm squares of foil, add a layer of pork fat and use the foil to smooth the edges into a nice shape, add the next slice of pork belly and finally the last layer of fat, drizzle liberally with the olive oil and season with sea salt flakes • Bake in the oven on a shallow baking tray, with the foil open, for 20–25 minutes until firmed up and crisp on the top

Make the crackling • Break the tofu skin or bean curd sheets into squares slightly larger than your pork belly pieces • Whisk the remaining ingredients (except the oil) in a bowl and dip in the curd squares • Heat the oil in a frying pan over a medium-high heat and shallow-fry the bean curd squares for 3–4 minutes until golden brown • Remove from the oil and drain on kitchen paper – they will crisp up once they dry out

Make the mash • Thinly slice the onions, peel and thinly slice the garlic, peel the potatoes and cut them into chunks • Heat the vegetable oil in the frying pan you used for cooking the crackling over a low heat then add the thinly sliced

FOR THE APPLE GRAVY
5 tbsp applesauce
1 tsp yeast extract
    (we use Marmite)
1 tsp cornflour
150ml vegetable stock

FOR THE WILTED KALE
1 tbsp plant-based butter
300g kale
sea salt

onions with a pinch of salt • Cook for about 25 minutes, stirring regularly and making sure they brown but do not burn • Add the garlic and cook for another 2 minutes then remove from the heat • Taste the onion and season to perfection – a little brown sugar could go a long way here • Meanwhile, bring a large saucepan of water to the boil, and add a pinch of salt and the potato chunks • Cover and simmer for 16–18 minutes until the potatoes are cooked through • Drain and shake well in a colander to remove moisture • Blitz the caramelised onions and garlic into a purée with the butter and milk in a blender or using a stick blender – or leave them chunky if you prefer the texture • Combine with the potatoes and mash into a smooth mash – you can use a hand blender or potato ricer to make it silky smooth if you wish • Add more butter for creaminess and salt and pepper to taste

Make the apple gravy • In a small saucepan over a low heat combine the applesauce, yeast extract and cornflour, slowly mixing into a thick paste • Gradually add the vegetable stock until you have a thin gravy consistency • Strain through a sieve or blend to a smooth consistency

Wilt the kale • Melt the butter in a saucepan over a high heat • Add the kale and a splash of water, season with salt, and cook until wilted while still retaining its green colour

To serve • Place the mash in the centre of a plate and form into an irregular brick shape with a flat top • Top with the kale • Gently place the pork belly on top and top with pieces of crackling • Repeat with the other serving • Drizzle the gravy around the mash or serve in a jug on the side

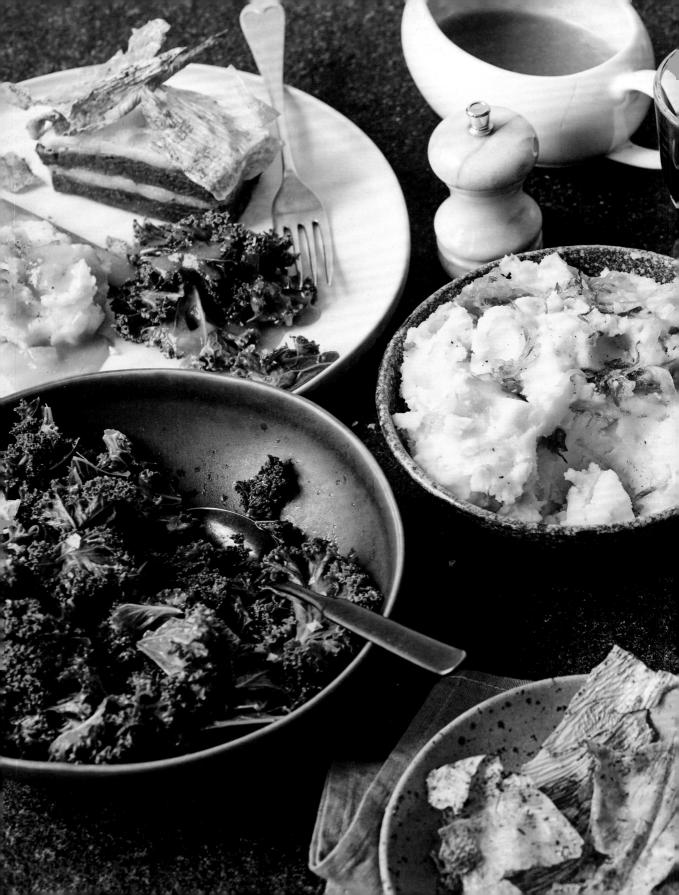

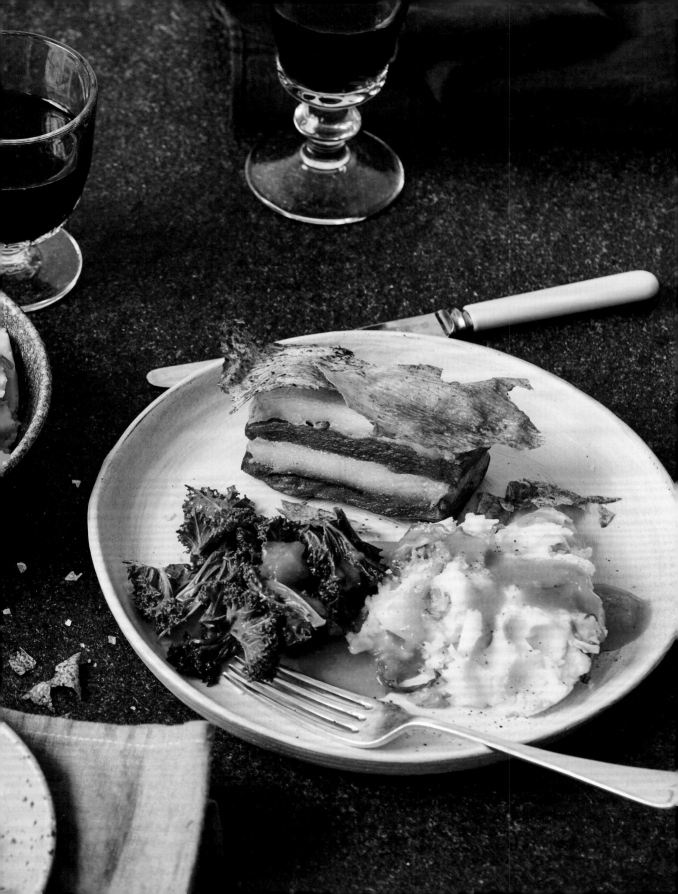

PORK GYOZA WITH ZIPPY DIPPY

If we see plant-based gyoza on the menu at a restaurant we order them, every time. We think they're delicious and, if you make this recipe, we think you'll think they're delicious too. They can be a little fiddly to make at first but, once you get the hang of it, you'll be bashing them out with no problem whatsoever. (Now's a great time to get some chopsticks if you haven't got them already.)

MAKES 32* (SERVES 4 AS A MAIN, 8 AS A SIDE)

FOR THE GYOZAS
225g napa cabbage or pointed sweetheart cabbage
2 spring onions, plus extra to serve
1 echalion shallot
2 garlic cloves
½ thumb-sized piece of ginger
225g plant-based pork mince
1 tsp caster sugar
¼ tsp ground white pepper
1 x pack gyoza dumpling wrappers (pot stickers)
1 tbsp sunflower oil
flaky sea salt

FOR THE ZIPPY DIPPY
120ml rice wine vinegar
60ml light soy sauce
1 tbsp chilli oil
¼ orange

Food processor (optional) • Fine grater or microplane • Pastry brush • Wide, deep frying pan with lid

*This recipe is enough to make 2 portions to freeze and 2 to eat straight away as a main • If you only want enough for 4 then halve the recipe

Prepare the gyoza ingredients • Thinly slice the cabbage • Put in a large bowl and sprinkle with a big pinch of flaky salt • Leave for 15 minutes, then squeeze the cabbage dry in a clean cloth • Trim and thinly slice the spring onions • Peel and finely dice the shallot and garlic • Peel and grate the ginger

Make the filling • In a large bowl, combine the pork mince, cabbage, most of the spring onions, shallot, garlic, ginger, sugar and a pinch of salt and the white pepper • Mix well, then use your hands to knead the mixture until it holds together • If you prefer a speedier food-processor method, blitz the cabbage to chop it into small pieces, then add the pork, spring onions, shallot, garlic, ginger and sugar and seasoning • Pulse so that the ingredients break down and everything mixes together • The vegetables will chop into finer pieces and the mince will break into the mixture, too • Spoon into a large bowl

Shape the gyozas • Fill a small bowl with cold water • Lay a dumpling wrapper on a board; dip a brush into the water and brush liberally around the edge • Holding it in the palm of one hand, use a teaspoon to spoon around 2 teaspoons of the mixture into the wrapper, then use both hands to pleat each side together to crimp the edges of the gyoza • Repeat with the rest of the mixture to make 32 pieces • Freeze any that you'd like to save for another time

Cook the gyozas • Heat 1 teaspoon of sunflower oil in a large, wide frying pan with a lid over a medium heat • Add the dumplings (base side down) and cook for about 2 minutes, until crispy and golden on the flat side (cook 8–10 gyoza at a time) • After 2 minutes, add a splash of water (100–120ml) to the pan • Cover and steam the dumplings for 3 minutes, then remove the lid and cook for another couple of minutes so they crisp up again • Repeat with the rest of the gyozas, with more oil as necessary, keeping the finished dumplings warm

Make the dipping sauce • Put the rice wine vinegar, light soy sauce and chilli oil in a bowl and mix together, adding a splash of orange juice to taste

Time to serve • Serve the dumplings on a large plate, with the dipping sauce alongside, and scatter with the remaining spring onions

NOTE
Treat frozen gyozas as above but use 150ml water and steam for 1 more minute before crisping up

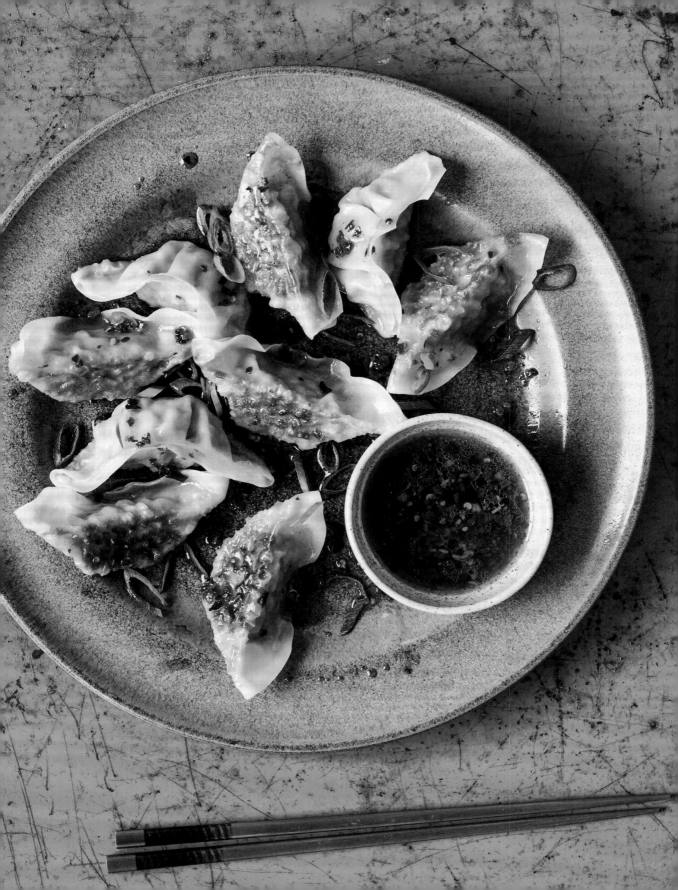

WEEPING TIGER JAY

One restaurant in London we visit very regularly is Busaba. There are a few branches across the city, and they specialise in Thai food. Their menu is really good but one dish we order all the time is Weeping Tiger Jay. It's rich and aromatic, it's got a fantastic robust texture and it works beautifully with rice. We love it so much we decided to make our own version for you to cook at home, just in case you don't live near a Busaba.

SERVES 2

FOR THE PORK
1 tbsp vegetable oil, plus
    2 tbsp to cook
2 tbsp dark soy sauce
1½ tbsp light brown sugar
2 tbsp plant-based fish
    sauce
¼ tsp ground black pepper
280g plant-based pork
    pieces
2 tbsp cornflour

FOR THE RICE
150g Thai jasmine rice
300ml cold water
1 jasmine tea bag
1 star anise
1 tsp fine sea salt

FOR THE SAUCE
1 tbsp cornflour
2 tbsp water, plus more to
    blend
1 red chilli
5–6 large Thai basil leaves
2 tbsp plant-based fish
    sauce
3 tbsp dark soy sauce or
    tamari
2 tbsp light brown sugar
½ tsp garlic powder
½ tsp ground ginger
½ tsp Chinese five-spice

FOR THE GARNISH
1 red chilli
1 spring onion
handful of fresh coriander
    or Thai basil leaves

FOR THE GREENS
150g spring greens or
    sweetheart cabbage
150g shiitake mushrooms
1 garlic clove
1 red chilli
1 tbsp vegetable oil
1 tbsp light soy sauce

1 medium saucepan • 1 small saucepan • 2 frying pans

Marinate the pork • Put the tablespoon of the vegetable oil in a bowl with the soy sauce, brown sugar, fish sauce and ground pepper and stir to combine • Add the pork pieces and fold to combine and coat • Set the bowl to one side

Cook the rice • Rinse the rice in a sieve under cold running water for 1 minute • Tip into a medium saucepan and pour over the cold water • Add the tea bag, star anise and salt and bring to the boil • Once boiling, reduce the heat to a low simmer, cover and cook for 12 minutes • After 12 minutes, when all the water has been absorbed by the rice, take the pan off the heat and leave the rice to rest with the lid on

Make the sauce • Mix the cornflour and water in a bowl to make a slurry • Deseed the red chilli and cut it into slithers • Pick the basil leaves and cut into long, thin pieces • Add the fish sauce, soy sauce or tamari, brown sugar, garlic powder, ground ginger and Chinese five-spice to a small saucepan and warm over a medium heat • Once the sauce is gently simmering, add the chilli and basil and stir for 1 minute before stirring in the cornflour slurry • Reduce the heat and simmer for 5–6 minutes

Prep the garnish • Trim and thinly slice the red chilli and spring onion at an angle • Pick the coriander leaves and finely chop, or pick the Thai basil leaves and leave whole

Prepare the greens • Destalk the greens and cut into thick ribbons • Thinly slice the shiitake mushrooms • Peel the garlic and thinly slice it widthways • Dice the red chilli • Heat the vegetable oil in a frying pan over a medium heat • Add the shiitake mushrooms and cook for 2–3 minutes • Add the garlic and chilli and cook for about 2 minutes until aromatic • Add the greens and soy sauce and cook for a minute or two until slightly wilted

Finish the pork • Transfer the marinated pork pieces to a mixing bowl and pour the remaining marinade into the pan with the sauce • Sprinkle the cornflour over the marinated pork pieces and stir to coat • Heat the 2 tablespoons of vegetable oil in a frying pan or wok over a medium heat • Add the marinated pork pieces and cook for 3–4 minutes until crispy • When the pieces are crispy, pour the sauce into the pan or wok and stir to coat

Time to serve • Fluff up the rice and spoon into serving bowls or plates along with the weeping tiger jay and stir-fried greens and bring to the table • Garnish with the chilli, spring onion, coriander and tuck in!

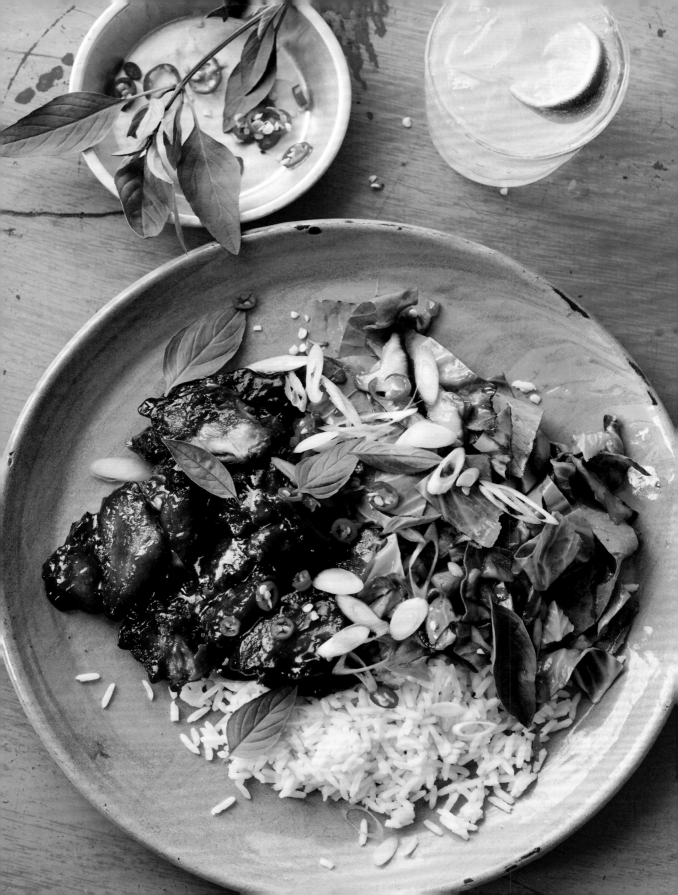

CHORIZO RISOTTO

A lot of people turn their noses up at risotto because they think it's bland and one-dimensional. We think that's a shame because risotto, when cooked well, is delicious. We played around with this recipe for quite a while, tweaking and altering it until we got it just right. We cook down red onions and cherry tomatoes before adding chunks of plant-based chorizo sausages spiced with paprika and fennel seeds. It's finished with a layer of soft rice and plant-based cream mixed through for the ultimate flavour sensation.

SERVES 4

FOR THE RISOTTO
2 red onions
3 garlic cloves
drizzle of olive oil
4 plant-based chorizo
    sausages (about 215g)
300g cherry tomatoes
1 tsp smoked paprika
1 tsp dried rosemary
1 tsp fennel seeds
1 tsp dried thyme
2 vegetable stock pots or
    cubes
1 litre boiling water
300g risotto rice
200ml plant-based cream
2 tbsp nooch (nutritional
    yeast)
½ lemon
sea salt and black pepper

TO SERVE
250g mixed leaves
thick balsamic vinegar
olive oil
handful of fresh basil leaves

Heavy-based saucepan • Heatproof jug

Prepare the risotto base • Peel and dice the red onions and garlic cloves • Place a heavy-based saucepan over a medium heat and add the drizzle of olive oil • Add the diced onion, garlic and a pinch of salt, mix well and cook for 5–10 minutes, or until the onions begin to soften

Cook the sausages • Cut the plant-based chorizo sausages into small chunks (removing any skin if necessary) and add to the pan • Mix well and cook according to the packet instructions (usually 10–15 minutes)

Prepare the tomatoes • Cut the cherry tomatoes in half and add to the pan with the paprika, dried rosemary, fennel seeds and dried thyme • Cook for 5 minutes until the cherry tomatoes break down and start to soften • Once the tomatoes are cooked, remove about a third of the tomato and sausage mixture from the pan and spoon it into a bowl (this is for the topping) • Leave to one side until needed

Cook the risotto • Mix the vegetable stock pots or cubes with the boiling water in a heatproof jug and mix well until completely dissolved • Add the rice to the pan and stir for 1 minute • Pour one third of the hot vegetable stock into the pan and mix well • Cook for 10 minutes, stirring frequently, before pouring another third of the stock into the pan • Cook for another 10 minutes, stirring frequently, before pouring in the rest of the stock and cooking for a final 10 minutes, or until the rice is soft and has absorbed all of the water but still has a bit of bite to it • When the risotto rice is tender and has absorbed all of the stock, mix through the plant-based cream and nooch • Squeeze in the lemon juice, catching any pips in your free hand • Cook for a minute or so until the cream and lemon juice is absorbed into the rice • Taste and season accordingly with salt and pepper

Make the salad • Dress the mixed leaves with a splash of balsamic vinegar and olive oil

Time to serve • Serve the risotto in bowls and top with a spoonful of the tomato mixture, some fresh basil leaves and pepper • Serve a large bowl of salad in the middle of the table and tuck in!

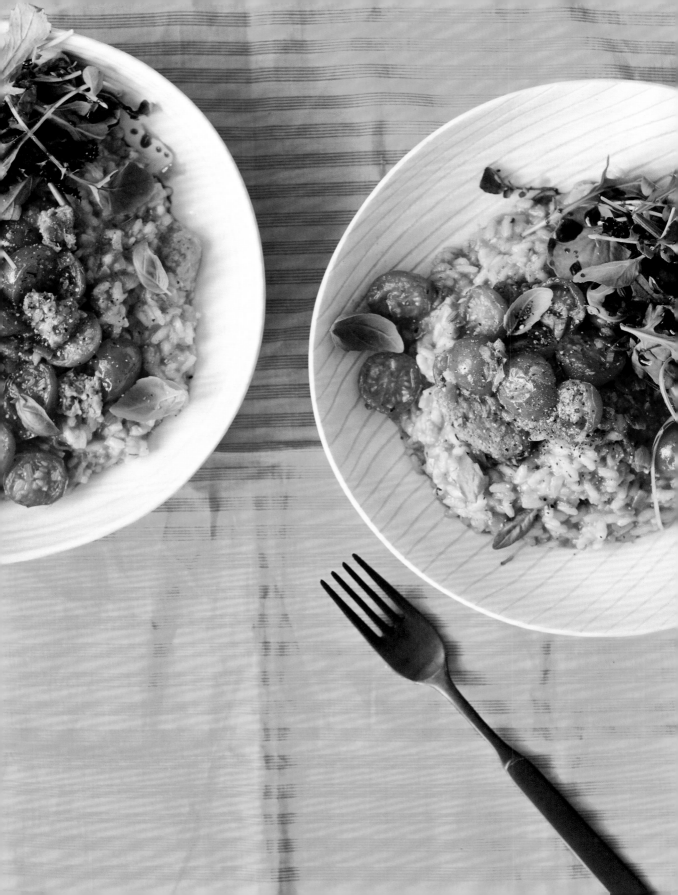

SARAH'S SUCCULENT SAUSAGE PASTA

This dish ticks all the boxes. It's meaty, saucy, flavourful and it doesn't take that long to make. We've made a fair few pasta dishes in our time, but this is right up there with the best. In fact, this is Ian's girlfriend Sarah's favourite pasta dish! The sauce is made from cooking down red onions until super soft before mixing them through sausage meat, sun-dried tomatoes and fennel seeds. We then stir through plant-based cream and sun-dried tomato pesto to create a sauce that coats the pasta perfectly. Give it a whirl, we bet you'll love it!

SERVES 4

Pestle and mortar • Large, deep saucepan • Large pot • Kettle boiled

FOR THE PASTA
2 red onions
6 plant-based Cumberland sausages
6 sun-dried tomatoes from a jar
1 tbsp fennel seeds
1 tsp black peppercorns
1 vegetable stock cube
400ml boiling water
2 tbsp olive oil
1 tbsp oil from the sun-dried tomato jar
4 tbsp sun-dried tomato pesto
450g dried pasta of your choice (we use rigatoni)
1 tbsp nooch (nutritional yeast), plus extra for sprinkling
1 tsp dried chilli flakes
100ml plant-based cream (ideally single)
sea salt

TO SERVE
handful of basil leaves
freshly ground black pepper

Prepare the ingredients • Peel and dice the red onions • Slice open the sausages and remove the 'skin' • Thinly slice the sun-dried tomatoes • Place the fennel seeds and peppercorns into a mortar and grind them to a powder with the pestle

Prepare the sauce • Mix the stock cube with the boiling water in a heatproof jug until dissolved • Place a large, deep saucepan over a medium-high heat and add the olive oil and sun-dried tomato oil • Once warm, add the diced red onion and a pinch of salt • Mix well and cook for 5–10 minutes, or until the onion softens • Once the onion softens, crumble in the sausage meat and stir for 4 minutes • After 4 minutes, add the ground pepper and fennel seeds to the pan and stir for a minute • Add the sun-dried tomatoes and stir for another few minutes • At this point, add the sun-dried tomato pesto and hot stock, mix well and bring to the boil, then reduce the heat and simmer for 10 minutes, or until all of the water has evaporated

While the sauce simmers, cook the pasta • Add a big pinch of salt to a large pot of boiling water over a medium heat, add the pasta and cook according to the packet instructions

Finish the dish • Mix the nooch, chilli flakes and cream through the sauce • Pick the basil leaves and finely chop • Once the pasta is cooked, spoon a ladleful of pasta water into the saucepan of sauce, stir to combine and turn off the heat • Drain the pasta in a colander and immediately transfer the pasta to the saucepan

Time to serve • Sprinkle half the basil over the pasta and stir the pasta into the sauce until well coated • Transfer the pasta into serving bowls, season with nooch and pepper, garnish with the remaining basil and serve immediately

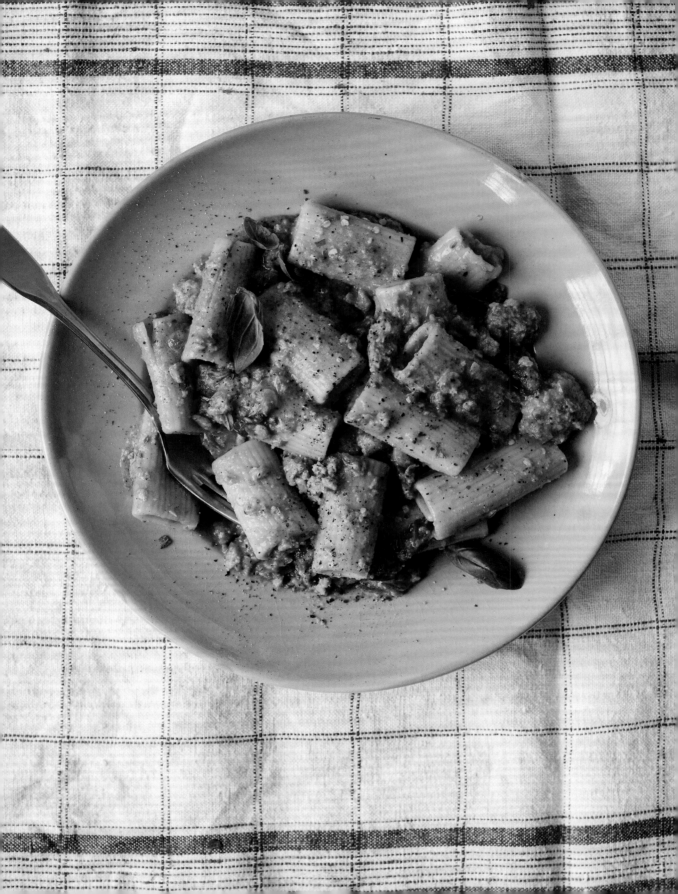

RACK 'O' RIBS

This is about as meaty as a vegetable can be; the bite on these bad boys is truly astonishing.

A few years ago, Derek Sarno introduced us to king oyster mushrooms and since then we've used them in dozens of recipes. Mushrooms are our absolute faves, and, if you feel the same, you should try these. They're trimmed to perfection before being skewered to one another to get a ridiculously meaty-rack-of-ribs look. The whole thing is then coated in a rich BBQ sauce and cooked to perfection to give you the ultimate showstopper – they really are knockout. Serve them with a slaw if you fancy a fresh accompaniment. (And chips, of course.)

SERVES 8 AS A SHARING DISH

FOR THE RIBS
16 king oyster mushrooms

FOR THE MARINADE
3 tbsp BBQ seasoning
6 tbsp olive oil
1 tbsp tamari
1 tbsp creamy tahini
2 tsp liquid smoke

FOR THE STICKY SAUCE
200g good-quality plant-based BBQ sauce
1 tbsp maple syrup
1 tbsp creamy tahini
1 tsp brown rice miso paste
1 tbsp tamari
1 tbsp apple cider vinegar
½ tbsp dried chilli flakes
sea salt and black pepper

FOR THE DIPPING SAUCE
100g good-quality plant-based BBQ sauce
1 tbsp tamari
1 tbsp sriracha
1 tbsp apple cider vinegar
sea salt and black pepper

Preheat oven to 200°C • 8 bamboo skewers • Large baking tray lined with foil • 2 extra-long BBQ metal skewers • Pastry brush

Prepare the mushrooms • Cut the top off the king oyster mushrooms and set to one side to use for another recipe • Trim any fatter mushroom stems to a thinner size so they match the thinner mushrooms

Marinate the mushrooms • Combine all the marinade ingredients in a large bowl • Add the mushroom stems and toss to coat

Skewer the mushrooms • Using a bamboo skewer, push one oyster mushroom stem lengthways down the skewer • Push down just over halfway and add another mushroom stem, lengthways, onto the skewer • Push down until they meet in the middle • Repeat this process until you have used all 8 skewers and you have 8 pairs of mushroom stems • Transfer the skewers onto a baking tray lined with foil and line them up so they are touching one another, creating a long line of mushrooms from the tallest to the shortest • Insert a large metal BBQ skewer into the left mushroom at the top of the line, closet to the edge touching the other mushroom • Push down the skewer so it goes through the whole line of mushrooms and connects them in a 'rib' – this will hold them all in place • Repeat with another long skewer and the other side of mushrooms

Cook the mushrooms • Place the tray of mushrooms in the oven to cook for 20 minutes, until the mushrooms soften

While the mushrooms cook, prepare the sticky sauce • Place all of the ingredients into a large bowl, season with salt and pepper and mix well until smooth

Brush the mushrooms with sauce • After 20 minutes, remove the mushrooms from the oven and place on a heatproof surface – if any of the marinade has burned at the bottom of the tray you can replace the foil with a new sheet • Use a pastry brush to brush all of the sticky sauce over the mushroom 'ribs', ensuring to get all around and between the mushroom stems • Place back in the oven for a final 20 minutes

Make the dipping sauce • Place all of the ingredients into a small bowl, season with salt and pepper and mix well until smooth • Spoon into a small serving bowl

Time to serve • Remove the ribs from the oven and serve with the dipping sauce on the side

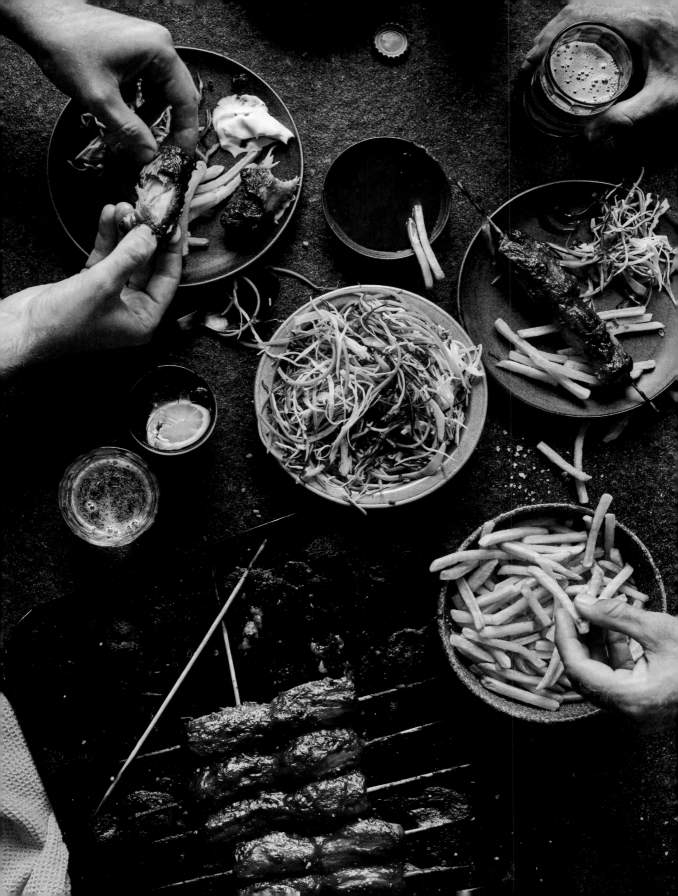

CHIPPY'S HOTTEST DOG

Chippy is Henry and EmJ's dog. She's a lovely little white Schnoodle and, if she could cook, we think she'd probably make a delicious hot dog slathered with gorgeous chilli. Don't let the 'hottest' put you off: these little beauties are spiced to the perfect heat with a combination of harissa and dried chilli flakes going into the lentil-based chilli – we then top with a final pinch of chilli flakes, but that depends how daring you're feeling. Also, here's something to ponder; when does hot dog stop being a sausage sandwich and when does a sausage sandwich start being a hot dog? Answers on a postcard...

Woof!

SERVES 6

FOR THE SPICY CHILLI

1 red onion
3 garlic cloves
drizzle of olive oil
2 x 400g tins green lentils
1 vegetable stock cube
200ml boiling water
1 tsp smoked paprika
1 tsp dried chilli flakes (or more if you like it extra spicy)
2 tbsp rose harissa paste
1 tbsp tomato purée
1 x 400g tin chopped tomatoes
2 tbsp smooth, runny almond butter
2 tbsp balsamic vinegar
1 tsp brown sugar
sea salt

FOR THE HOT DOGS

6 plant-based hot dog sausages
6 hot dog buns

TO SERVE

plant-based butter, for spreading
sriracha mayo, to taste
handful of plant-based grated cheese
3 tbsp crispy fried onions
small jar of sliced green jalapeños
black pepper (or more chilli flakes if you like it extra spicy)

Large saucepan

Make the chilli • Peel and dice the onion and garlic • Place a large saucepan over a medium heat and add the drizzle of olive oil • Once warm, add the diced onion, garlic and a pinch of salt • Mix well and cook for 5–10 minutes, or until the onion softens • While the onion and garlic are cooking, drain the lentils • Mix the stock cube with the boiling water in a heatproof jug until completely dissolved • Once the onion and garlic are soft, add the paprika, mix well and cook for a few seconds before adding the chilli flakes, harissa paste, tomato purée, drained lentils, tinned tomatoes, almond butter, balsamic vinegar, brown sugar and stock • Mix well, reduce the heat and simmer for 25–30 minutes while you make the rest of the dish – if the mixture becomes too thick, stir through a dash of water

Cook the hot dogs • Cook the hot dog sausages according to the packet instructions

Assemble the hot dogs • Taste and season the chilli • Toast and butter the hot dog buns (you can use a griddle pan if you want them to have char marks) and place each onto a serving plate, stretching them open wide • Place a cooked hot dog in each of the buns • Spoon a large spoonful of the chilli over the top of each sausage

Time to serve • Squeeze zig-zag lines of sriracha mayo over the top of the hot dogs • Scatter the hot dogs with grated cheese, crispy fried onions, sliced jalapeños and pepper before serving

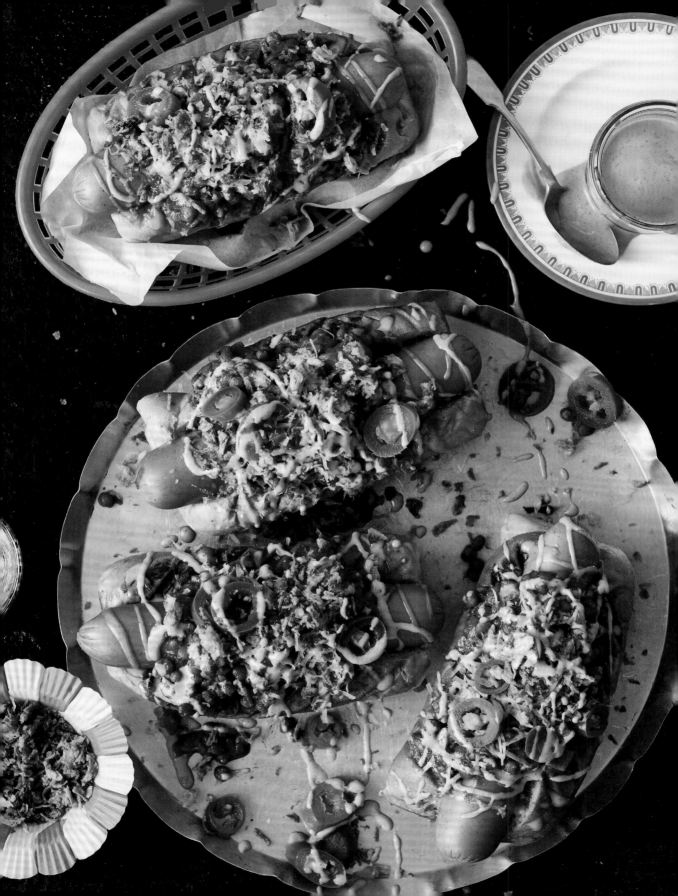

SAUSAGE AND STUFFING PASTRY PUFFS

Sausage rolls are good, but Sausage and Stuffing Pastry Puffs are even better. Meaty sausage, herby stuffing and sweet cranberry sauce all wrapped up in a crispy golden pastry pyramid. Your Christmas party snack platter just got a boost. These little guys couldn't be easier to make during a busy festive period – they only need a handful of ingredients, a baking tray and a short time in the oven until you get the perfect crispy snack.

MAKES 12

FOR THE SAUSAGE AND STUFFING
6 plant-based sausages (about 270g)
1 x 170g pack sage & onion stuffing
1 tbsp plant-based butter
2 tsp Dijon mustard
sea salt

FOR THE PASTRY PUFFS
2 x 320g ready-rolled plant-based puff pastry sheets
1 x 200g block plant-based cheese
1 x 250g jar good-quality cranberry sauce

FOR THE TOPPING
4 tbsp oat milk
½ tsp English mustard powder
black sesame seeds, for sprinkling

Small ramekin • 2 baking trays lined with baking parchment • Pastry brush • Small saucepan

Prepare the sausage and stuffing • Use a knife to slice the sausages in half and remove the meat from the 'skin' • Place the sausage meat into a medium bowl and mash with a fork • In a separate large mixing bowl or baking tray, make up the stuffing according to the packet instructions • Once the stuffing is cooked, and while it's still hot, add the butter to a bowl and mix well • Add the mashed sausage meat and Dijon mustard • Mix well and set aside to cool

Prepare the pastry and cheese • Roll one of the pastry sheets out on a board, keeping the pastry on the paper, with the longest edge horizontal • Using a knife, cut the sheet into 6 even squares – do this by cutting the sheet in half horizontally, then making two cuts, evenly spaced apart lengthways, to make the six squares • Repeat with the second sheet of pastry • Cut the block of cheese into 12 small even squares • Preheat oven to 200°C

Make the parcels • Place a square of cheese in the middle of each pastry square, positioning it diagonally so the points of the squares are at a different angle to the pastry square edges • Spoon a teaspoon of the cranberry sauce on top of each square of cheese • Weigh about 70g of the sausage mixture into a small ramekin, then tip out onto the cranberry sauce • Flatten the sausage mixture slightly with your hand • Continue to do this five more times until you've covered each square of cheese and chutney • Take each corner of the pastry square and bring them to the top of the stuffing, making all of the pastry corners meet at the top • Pinch the corners together well to ensure they are sealed • Repeat with the remaining pastry and filling until you have 12 parcels • Place the pastry puffs on 2 baking trays lined with baking parchment

Cook the sausage puffs • In a small bowl, mix together the oat milk and mustard powder • Brush all of the parcels with the milk mixture, ensuring all of the pastry is covered • Sprinkle the tops with black sesame seeds • Bake in the oven for 25–30 minutes, or until golden and crispy, turning the trays halfway through

Time to serve • Serve warm, but not straight out of the oven!

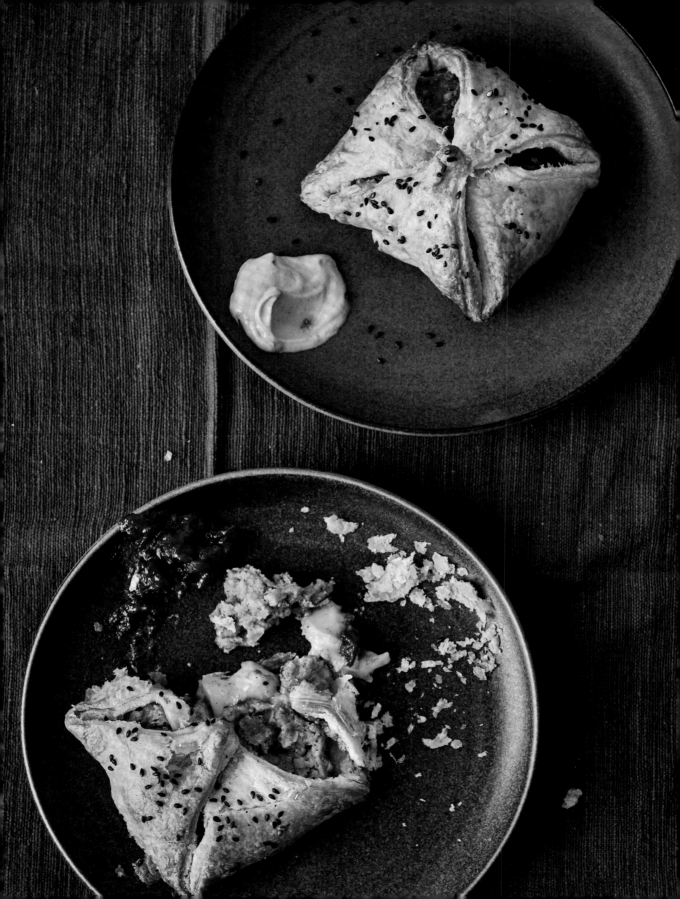

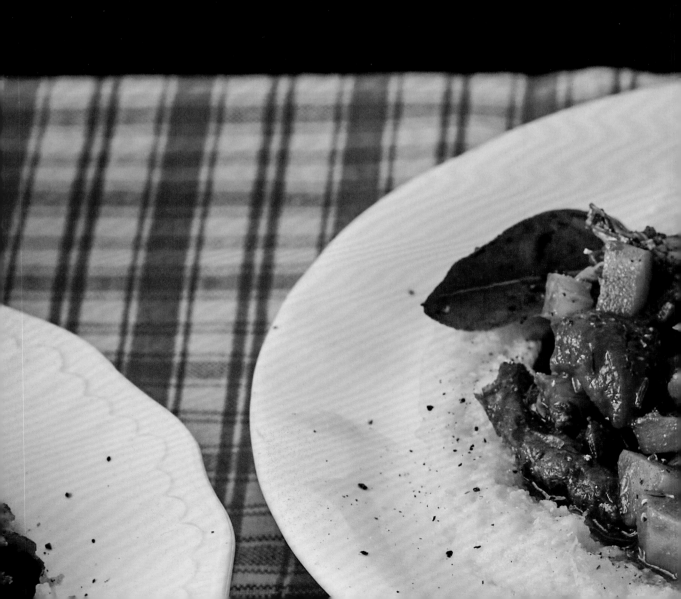

LAMB

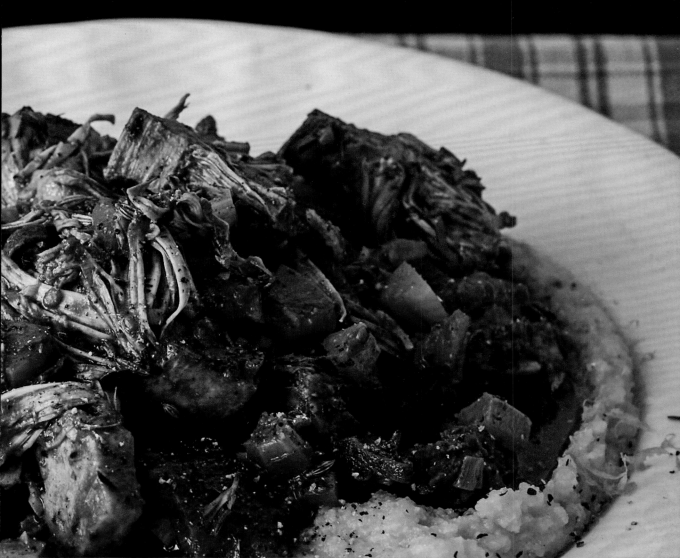

HARISSA-SPICED PULLED LAMB WITH GIANT COUSCOUS AND FETA SALAD

When it comes to heartiness, some salads just don't cut it: they might be delicious but you couldn't have them for your tea because they wouldn't fill you up – you'd end up needing a few biscuits or a slice of cake before bed to stave off guttural murmurings. This salad is different though. This salad will fill you up. This is a salad you could, and should, have for your tea. Pulled jackfruit coated in a harissa-spiced date rub and roasted to perfection, served with a giant couscous salad filled with crunchy toasted almonds and fresh herbs, drizzled with a fresh mint yoghurt to bring everything together.

SERVES 4

FOR THE LAMB
150g pitted dates
100g plant-based butter
drizzle of olive oil
2 tbsp mint jelly
1 tbsp ras el hanout
2 tsp rose harissa paste
2 garlic cloves
2 x 400g tins jackfruit
  in water
500g oyster mushrooms
sea salt and black pepper

FOR THE COUSCOUS SALAD
1 vegetable stock cube
300ml boiling water
drizzle of olive oil
200g giant couscous
100g toasted skin-on
  almonds
5 spring onions
15g fresh flat-leaf parsley
15g fresh coriander
15g fresh mint
100g pomegranate seeds
1 lemon
100g plant-based
  feta cheese
sea salt and black pepper

FOR THE MINT YOGHURT
a few fresh mint leaves
150g plain plant-based
  yoghurt
2 tbsp mint jelly
pinch of sea salt
1 lemon

Preheat oven to 180°C • Powerful blender • Deep baking dish • Large saucepan

Make the lamb • If the dates feel hard, place them in a heatproof bowl, cover with boiling water and leave to soak for 5 minutes • After 5 minutes, drain the water and spoon the dates into a powerful blender • Add the butter, olive oil, mint jelly, ras el hanout, harissa, peeled garlic cloves and a pinch of salt • Blend until the mixture forms a smooth, thick paste • Drain the jackfruit and place into a deep baking dish • Pull the oyster mushrooms using your hands and add them to the baking dish • Add the paste and mix really well until all of the jackfruit and mushrooms are coated in the paste • Cook in the oven for 30 minutes, or until the jackfruit feels really tender

Make the couscous salad • Mix the stock cube with the boiling water in a heatproof jug • Place a large saucepan over a medium heat and add a drizzle of olive oil • Add the giant couscous and toast for 2 minutes then pour in the stock • Bring to the boil and simmer for 8 minutes, or until the couscous feels cooked and has absorbed all of the water • Roughly chop the almonds, trim and thinly slice the spring onions and finely chop all of the herbs • Once the couscous has finished cooking, spoon into a large bowl • Mix through most of the chopped almonds, spring onions, chopped herbs and pomegranate seeds • Halve the lemon and squeeze in some juice, catching any pips in your free hand • Add a drizzle of olive oil and crumble in the plant-based feta (saving a little of everything for the top) • Taste and season with salt and pepper

Make the mint yoghurt • Thinly slice the mint leaves • Put the yoghurt in a small bowl and mix through the mint jelly, chopped mint leaves and salt • Halve the lemon and squeeze in the juice, catching any pips in your free hand • Spoon into a small serving bowl

Pull the lamb • Once the lamb is cooked, remove from the oven and pull the jackfruit into thin strips using two forks • Mix well until all of the jackfruit and mushrooms are coated in the sauce

Time to serve • Spoon the couscous salad into a large serving dish • Pile the pulled jackfruit and mushrooms on top of the salad or just to the side • Drizzle over some of the mint yoghurt and serve the rest in a small bowl on the side • Top all of the salad with any leftover herbs, pomegranate seeds and plant-based feta and sprinkle with freshly ground black pepper

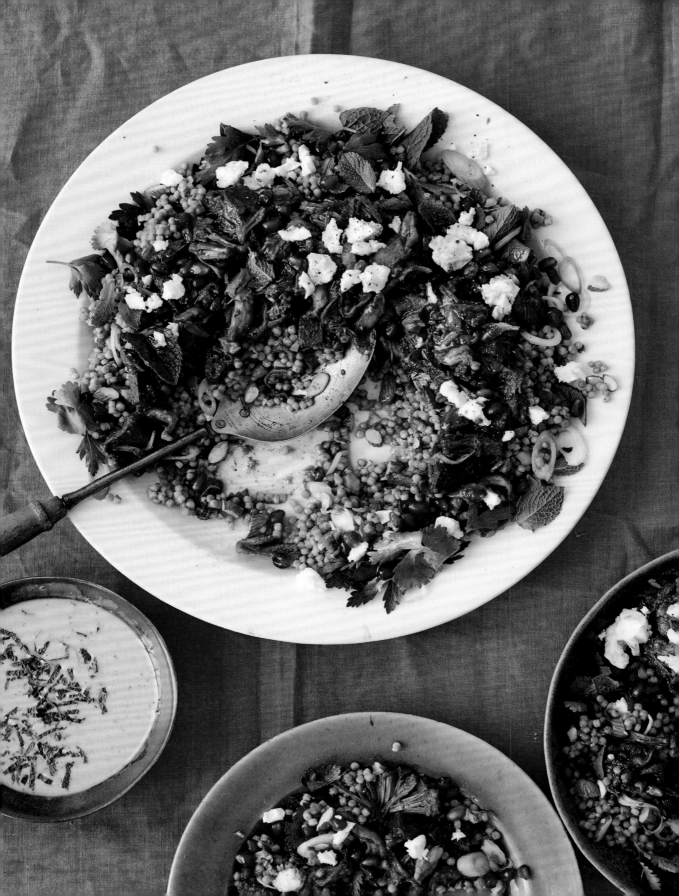

KASHMIRI LAMB WITH DUM ALOO AND NIGELLA NAAN

Curry, wonderful curry, how we love you so. So versatile, so variable, so very, very delicious. Saucy curries are fantastic but every so often a curry that's a little drier really hits the spot. This curry, goodness gracious, it REALLY hits the spot. As for those potatoes, don't get us started...

SERVES 4

FOR THE NIGELLA NAAN

310g white self-raising flour, plus extra for dusting
1 tsp sea salt
250g plain plant-based yoghurt
1 tsp nigella seeds
1 tsp sesame seeds
vegetable oil, for cooking

FOR THE ROASTED LAMB

2 x 400g tins young green jackfruit in water
2 tbsp rapeseed oil
1 tbsp garam marsala
1½ tsp ground turmeric
½ tsp cayenne pepper
½ tsp asafoetida
2 tsp sea salt

FOR THE CURRY PASTE

3 tbsp coriander seeds
2 tbsp cumin seeds
1 tbsp fenugreek seeds
seeds from 4 green cardamom pods
2 cinnamon sticks
1 tbsp basmati rice
3 tbsp raw unsalted cashews
200ml water

FOR THE DUM ALOO

1kg baby potatoes
3 tsp sea salt
2 tbsp vegetable oil or vegetable shortening
1 tsp garam masala
1 tsp cayenne pepper
1 tsp turmeric

Preheat oven to 220°C • 2 roasting trays • 2 frying pans • Powerful blender • Saucepan • Rolling pin • Tongs

Make the naan dough • Put the flour, salt, yoghurt, nigella seeds and sesame seeds in a bowl and stir to combine • Set aside for later

Prepare the roasted lamb • Drain, rinse and pat dry the jackfruit • Put the oil, garam masala, turmeric, cayenne, asafoetida and salt in a bowl and stir to combine • Add the jackfruit to the bowl and fold to cover and coat • Spread the jackfruit out on a roasting tray, put the tray in the oven and roast for 30–35 minutes until the jackfruit is nice and dry

Prepare the curry paste • Put the coriander seeds, cumin seeds, fenugreek seeds, cardamom seeds, cinnamon sticks and rice in a dry frying pan and toast over a low heat for 2–3 minutes, stirring frequently so they don't burn, until fragrant • Leave the spices to cool, then add them to a powerful blender with the cashews and blitz into a fine powder • Add the water to the blender and blitz into a paste

Prepare the potatoes for the dum aloo • Put the potatoes in a saucepan with 2 teaspoons of the salt, cover with water, bring to the boil then simmer for 15–17 minutes until tender • Drain the potatoes and shake in a colander to chuff them up • Add the potatoes to a roasting tray along with the oil or shortening, remaining teaspoon of salt, garam masala, cayenne and turmeric • Put the tin in the oven and roast the potatoes for 30 minutes (at the same oven temperature as the jackfruit) to crisp them up a little

Prepare the dum aloo sauce • Peel and thinly slice the onion, garlic and ginger • Destem and thinly slice the chillies • Warm the oil in a frying pan (the same pan you used for the spices) over a low heat, add the onion, garlic, ginger, chilli and salt and cook for 8–10 minutes until soft and caramelised • Add the curry paste you made earlier and fry for a minute or two, then add the yoghurt, turmeric, tomato purée, sugar and tinned tomatoes and simmer for 10 minutes

Cook the naans • Split the dough into 4 pieces • Lightly dust a work surface with flour and roll out the dough into naans about 5mm thick • Warm a little oil in a frying pan over a medium heat, add a naan to the pan and fry for 3–4 minutes on each side until golden and slightly charred in patches, turning them with tongs • Repeat with the remaining naans

FOR THE DUM ALOO SAUCE

1 onion
8 garlic cloves
40g piece of fresh ginger
3 fresh hot green chillies
2 tbsp vegetable oil
1 tsp sea salt
2 tbsp plain plant-based yoghurt
1 tsp turmeric
2 tbsp tomato purée
1 tsp light brown sugar
1 x 400g tin chopped tomatoes

TO SERVE

30g fresh coriander
1 lemon
plain plant-based yoghurt
crispy fried onions

Time to serve • Pick and finely chop the coriander leaves • Finely chop half the coriander stalks • Halve the lemon • Sprinkle the coriander stalks over the lamb, squeeze over half the lemon juice (catching any pips in your free hand) and fold to combine • Transfer the potatoes to the sauce and fold to coat • Taste everything and season to perfection • Transfer the lamb and dum aloo to serving bowls, plate up the naan, bring to the table and serve with the coriander, yoghurt and crispy fried onions

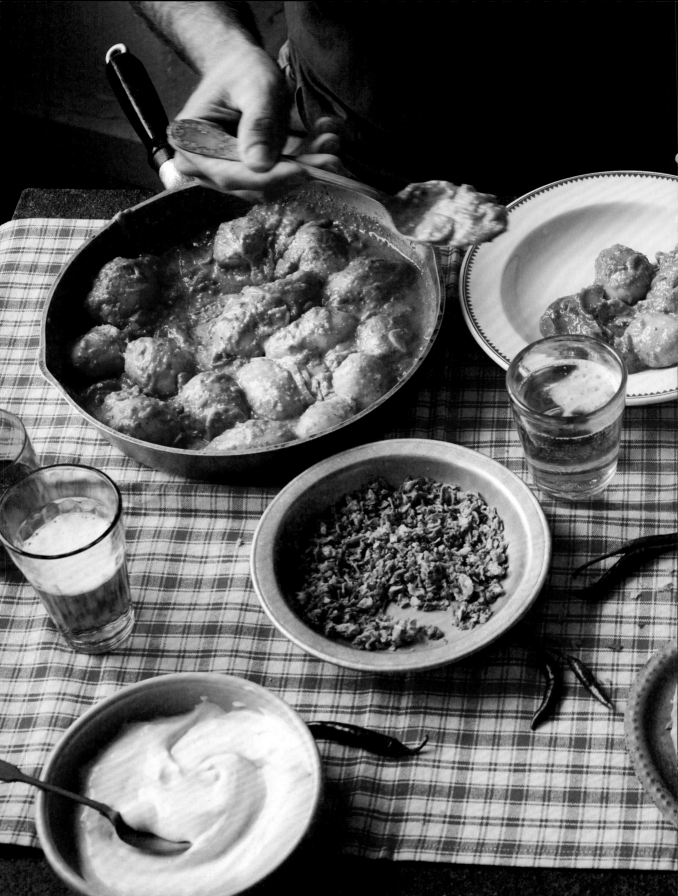

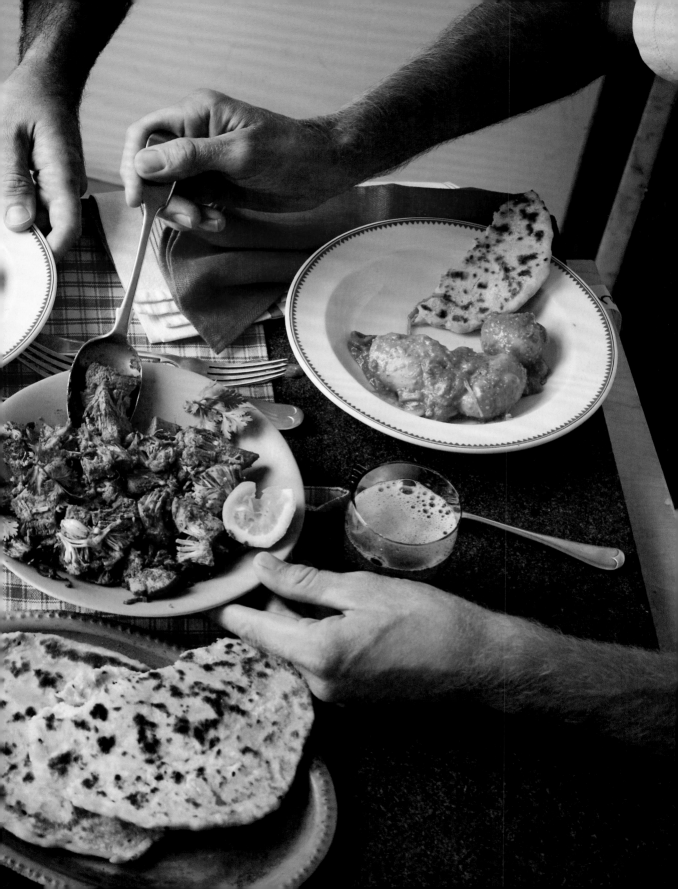

LUSCIOUS LAMB RAGU WITH SILKY POLENTA

Polenta. It's kinda like porridge, it's kinda like custard and, if you cook it well, it's kinda like liquid gold. If you're not convinced by polenta, allow us to change your mind because this is, without question, one of the tastiest recipes in this book. You can thank us later...

SERVES 6–8

FOR THE MEAT
2 x 400g tins young green
    jackfruit in water
200g oyster mushrooms
8 plant-based sausages
3 tbsp olive oil
3 tbsp Italian dried herbs
2 tsp fennel seeds
1 tsp dried chilli flakes
2 tsp sea salt
pinch of ground black
    pepper

FOR THE SAUCE
1 large onion
2 carrots
4 garlic cloves
2 celery sticks
20g fresh sage leaves
4 tbsp olive oil
3 fresh bay leaves
2 tsp sea salt
1 tsp dried chilli flakes
100ml plant-based
    white wine
1 tsp cacao powder
2 tbsp tomato purée
2 tbsp maple syrup
2 tbsp light soy sauce
1 x 400g tin plum tomatoes
400ml water

FOR THE POLENTA
2 litres oat milk
1 tsp sea salt
400g polenta
150g plant-based butter or
    vegetable shortening
1 lemon
200g grated plant-based
    cheddar
4 tbsp nooch (nutritional
    yeast)

TO SERVE
fresh flat-leaf parsley
nooch (nutritional yeast) or
    plant-based parmesan,
    for sprinkling
drizzle of extra-virgin olive oil

Preheat oven to 220°C • Roasting tray • Large heavy-based saucepan • Large saucepan • Whisk • Fine grater or microplane

Prepare the meat • Wash, drain and pat dry the jackfruit • Put the jackfruit in a roasting tray and crush the chunks in between your fingers to split the fibres • Remove any seeds (they look a little like cannellini beans) • Chop the mushrooms and sausages into similar-sized chunks and add them to the tray • Drizzle over the olive oil, sprinkle with the herbs, fennel seeds and chilli flakes, salt and pepper and stir everything together • Roast in the oven for 30 minutes

Prepare the sauce • Peel and dice the onion, carrots and garlic and dice the celery • Pick and thinly slice the sage leaves • Warm the oil in a large heavy-based saucepan over a medium heat • Add the onion, carrots, celery and garlic, and cook, stirring, for 2 minutes • Add the sage, bay leaves, salt and chilli flakes to the pan, reduce the heat a little, stir to combine and sweat for 12–15 minutes • Add the wine, cacao powder, tomato purée, maple syrup, soy sauce, tomatoes, water and the roasted ingredients and simmer for 45 minutes–1 hour, breaking up the tomatoes with a wooden spoon, until the ragu is thick and silky

Prepare the polenta • Put the oat milk and salt in a large saucepan and bring to the boil • Slowly pour the polenta into the pan in a steady stream, whisking all the time • Turn the heat down to low and continue whisking every few minutes until the polenta is cooked through (follow the packet instructions – it should be thick and silky; if the polenta is too thick, add a splash more oat milk or water to loosen it) • Remove from the heat and add the butter or shortening, grate in the zest of the lemon, add the cheese and nooch and whisk until smooth • Taste and season to perfection

Time to serve • Finely chop some parsley • Spoon the polenta into bowls, top with the ragu, sprinkle over a little parsley, parmesan or nooch and finish with a drizzle of extra-virgin olive oil

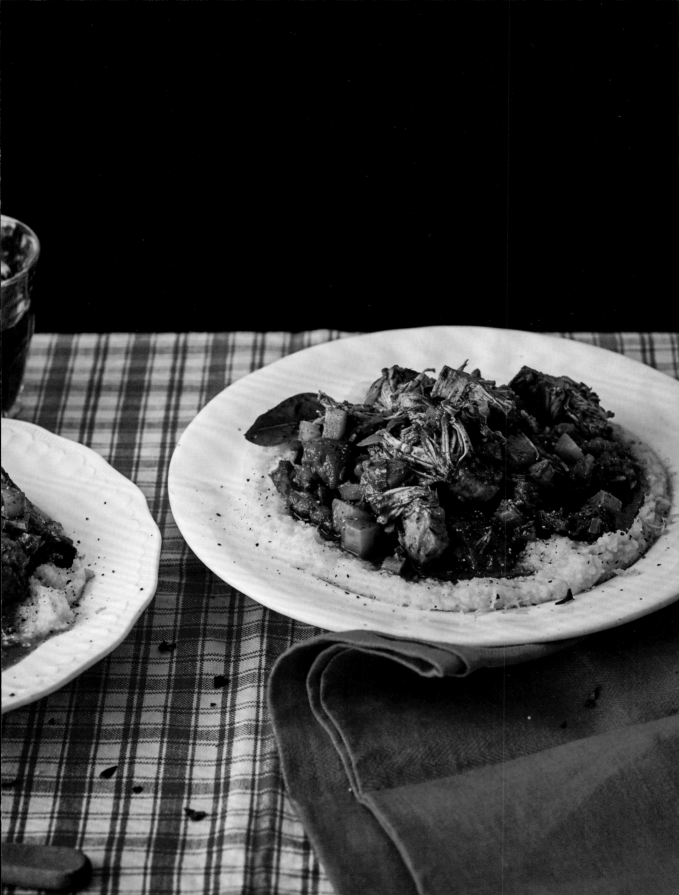

ISKENDER KEBAB WITH SPICED TOMATO SAUCE

Bread is usually used to mop up sauce but in this recipe the sauce is served on top of the bread. This dish hails from Turkey and we're big, big fans. Interesting textures and zippy, out-there flavours combine to create a truly delicious dish that you and your family will be pleased you cooked!

SERVES 4

FOR THE AUBERGINE
2 aubergines
drizzle of olive oil
sea salt

FOR THE LAMB
1 onion
5 garlic cloves
2 x 400g tins jackfruit
   in water
3 tbsp olive oil
3 tbsp tomato purée
2 tbsp ground coriander
2 tbsp ground cumin
1 lemon
salt

**FOR THE SPICED
TOMATO SAUCE**
1 onion
drizzle of olive oil
1 tsp smoked sweet paprika
1 tsp ground allspice
1 tbsp tomato purée
1 x 400g tin chopped
   tomatoes
1 tsp light brown sugar
100ml water
sea salt

FOR THE LAMB SAUCE
1 tbsp yeast extract (we use
   Marmite)
50ml hot water
15g fresh mint leaves
2 tbsp maple syrup
2 tbsp light soy sauce
2 tsp dried oregano
1 tsp cayenne pepper
2 tbsp plain plant-based
   yoghurt
½ tsp cacao powder
sea salt and black pepper

FOR THE PITTA BASE
4 pittas
olive oil, for drizzling
sea salt

Preheat oven to 200°C • 2 baking trays • Large saucepan • Hand blender • Powerful blender

Prepare the ingredients • Halve the aubergines lengthways and place on a baking tray cut side up • Drizzle with olive oil, sprinkle with a pinch of salt and cook in the oven for 40 minutes until completely soft • After 40 minutes, remove the aubergines from the oven and place to one side to cool down • Meanwhile, peel and dice the onion and garlic for the lamb • Drain the jackfruit, pat it dry and place it in a large baking tray, add the olive oil, tomato purée, the ground spices, a pinch of salt and the diced garlic and onion • Halve the lemon, squeeze in the juice from both halves (catching any pips in your free hand) and mix well until everything comes together • Cook in the oven for 30 minutes

Make the spiced tomato sauce • Peel and dice the onion • Heat the olive oil in a large saucepan over a medium heat • Add the diced onion and a pinch of salt, mix well and cook for 5–10 minutes, or until the onion softens • Mix through spices and cook for a couple of seconds, then add the tomato purée, tinned tomatoes, sugar and water • Bring to the boil then reduce the temperature and cook for 20 minutes • After 20 minutes, remove from the heat and use a hand blender to blend the mixture until smooth

Pull the aubergines • Once the aubergines are cooled, use a fork to pull all of the flesh from the inside (discarding the skins) and make thin strands in a pulled meat-like consistency

Mix the lamb sauce ingredients • Spoon the pulled aubergine into the baking tray with the cooked jackfruit • Put the yeast extract in a small bowl and mix with the hot water until completely dissolved • Finely chop the mint leaves and add to the baking tray, along with the yeast extract mixture and the rest of the lamb sauce ingredients • Mix well until everything comes together • Taste and season with salt and pepper

Mix the pitta base • Rip the pittas in half and place all of the halves on a baking tray • Drizzle the pittas with olive oil and sprinkle with some salt • Bake in the oven for 5 minutes until golden • Once cooked, remove from the oven and place to one side until needed

Make the tahini yoghurt • Peel the garlic and put in a powerful blender along with the yoghurt and tahini • Halve the lemon and squeeze in the juice from both halves (catching any pips in your free hand) and add the salt • Blend until smooth and creamy

**FOR THE TAHINI
YOGHURT**
1 garlic clove
270g plain plant-based
   yoghurt
115g creamy tahini
1 lemon
pinch of sea salt

**TO SERVE (ALL
OPTIONAL)**
handful each of fresh
   parsley and mint
drizzle of pomegranate
   molasses
sprinkle of toasted pine
   nuts
pickled green chillies

Assemble the dishes • Arrange all of the components in layers across
4 serving plates – start each plate with two halves of toasted pitta, top
each with a quarter of the lamb mixture and spoon over a good amount
of the tomato sauce before drizzling with tahini yoghurt

Time to serve • Finely chop the fresh herbs • Drizzle a small amount
of pomegranate molasses over each plate before topping with chopped
herbs, pine nuts and pickled green chillies

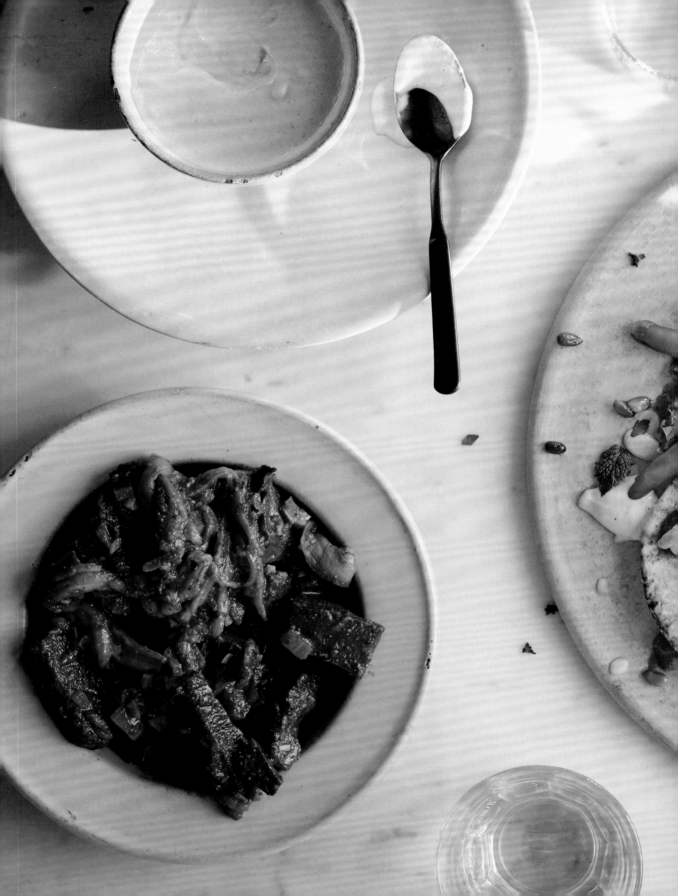

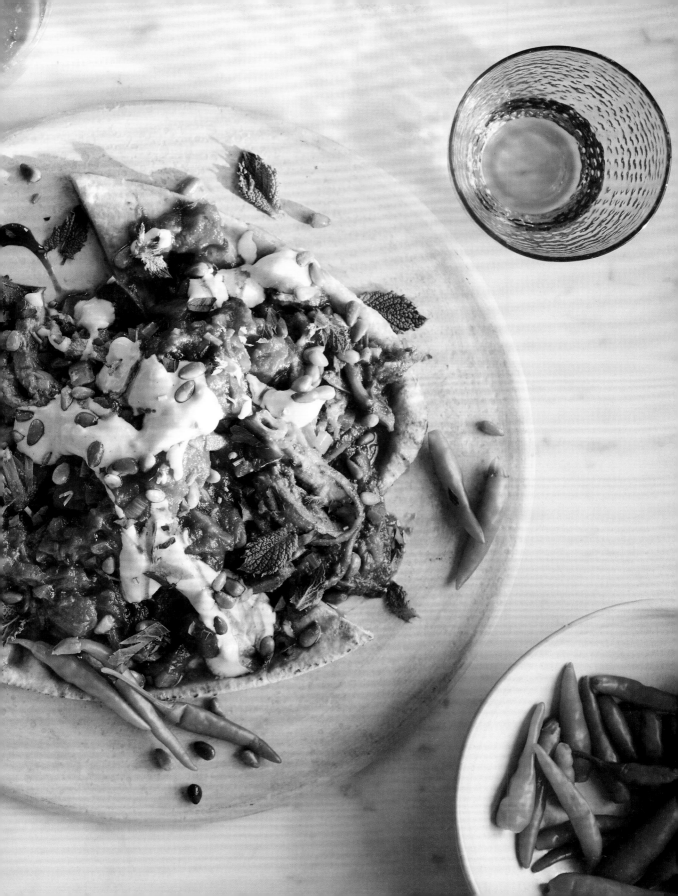

LANCASHIRE HOTPOT

What's the best thing to come out of Lancashire? The road to Yorkshire. (Sorry, couldn't resist.) In all seriousness, we love Lancashire. It's a county that's produced more than its fair share of great things and the Lancashire Hotpot is one of them. Potato dauphinoise meets plant-based lamb casserole – the base for this dish is a rich, hearty stew spiced with bay leaves, rosemary and mint jelly, topped with crispy thin potatoes sprinkled with nooch (nutritional yeast) to bring it all together. Easy on the eye, rich flavours and warming satisfaction. It's the perfect replacement for a full roast dinner on a Sunday afternoon.

SERVES 4

FOR THE TOPPING
1kg Maris Piper potatoes
1–2 tbsp nooch (nutritional yeast)
drizzle of olive oil
sea salt flakes

FOR THE BASE
240g baby carrots
drizzle of olive oil
1 x 400g tin jackfruit in water
1 x pack plant-based beef chunks (about 300g)
1 tbsp mint jelly
2 onions
2 celery sticks
3 garlic cloves
500ml boiling water
1 plant-based OXO cube
1 vegetable stock cube
2 rosemary sprigs
2 thyme sprigs
3 bay leaves
2 tbsp tomato purée
2–3 tsp yeast extract (we use Marmite)
1 tbsp Henderson's relish
sea salt and black pepper

FOR THE GREENS
80g plant-based butter
200g tenderstem broccoli
100g frozen peas
200g sliced spring greens
1 lemon
pinch of sea salt
50g toasted pine nuts

Preheat oven to 190°C • 2 large saucepans • Baking tray • Large casserole dish

Prepare and part-cook the potatoes • Cut the potatoes into 3mm-thick slices (no need to peel) • Place into a large saucepan of salted water and bring to the boil • Reduce the heat and cook for 3–4 minutes until tender but still holding their shape • Drain and set aside

Prepare the carrots and roast the meat • Halve the carrots lengthways • Put the carrots on a baking tray, drizzle with olive oil and season • Mix to coat and cook in the oven for 5–10 minutes until they begin to soften • After 5 minutes, remove the tray from the oven • Drain and rinse the jackfruit and mix it through the carrots, add the plant-based beef, mint jelly and another drizzle of oil (if needed) • Mix and return to the oven for 30 minutes until the carrots soften

Make the base • Peel and thinly slice the onions, trim and dice the celery and peel and dice the garlic • Place a large casserole dish over a medium heat and add a splash of olive oil • Add the onions, celery, garlic and a pinch of salt • Mix well and cook for 5–10 minutes until the onions begin to soften • Pour the boiling water into a heatproof jug, crumble in the OXO and stock cubes and stir until dissolved • Pick the rosemary and thyme leaves • Pour the stock into the casserole dish and mix through the rosemary, thyme, bay leaves, tomato purée, yeast extract and Henderson's relish • Bring to the boil, then reduce the heat and simmer for 15 minutes

Finish the topping • Increase the oven temperature to 220°C • Once the stew has simmered for 15 minutes and reduced a little, mix through the roasted jackfruit, plant-based beef and carrots • Taste and season lightly • Arrange the part-cooked potato slices over the top, layering them neatly • Sprinkle with some nooch, sea salt flakes and drizzle over some olive oil • Cook in the oven for 10–15 minutes, or until the potatoes turn crispy and golden on top

Cook the greens • Place a large saucepan over a medium heat (you can use the pan you used to cook the potatoes) and add the butter • Add the greens and mix well • Cover and cook for 10 minutes until the spring greens have wilted • Halve the lemon and squeeze in some juice, catching any pips with your free hand • Add the salt and the pine nuts

Time to serve • Remove the hotpot from the oven and serve in the middle of the table • Spoon the greens into a serving bowl and serve alongside

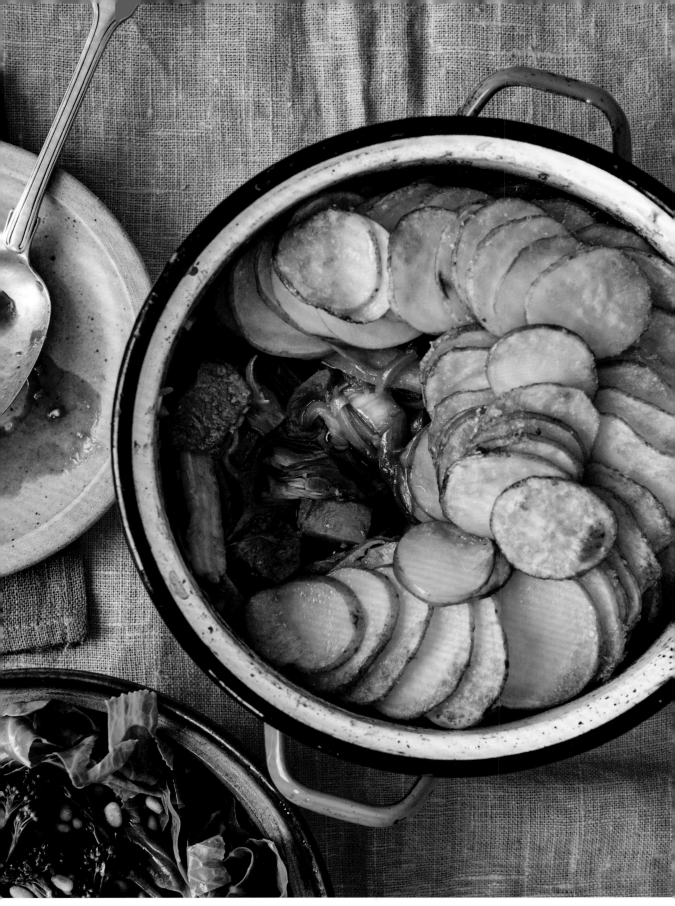

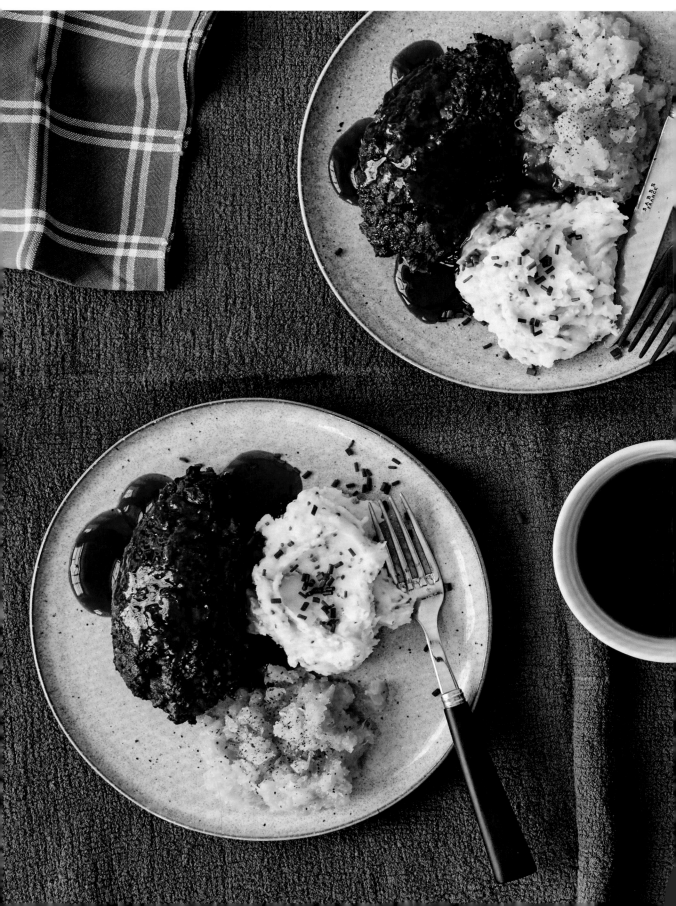

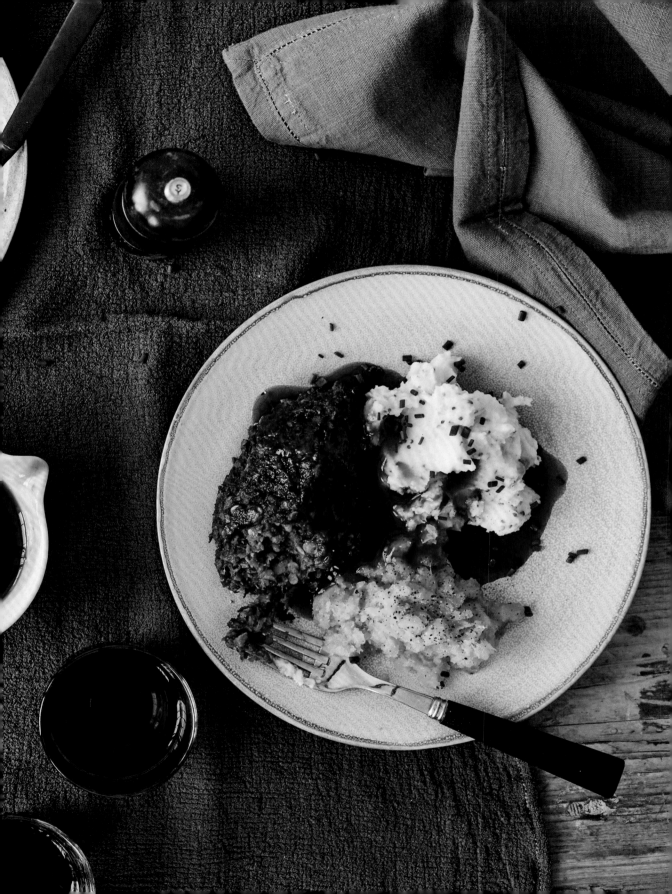

YEMISTA (GREEK STUFFED PEPPERS) WITH EASY TZATZIKI

We started BOSH! over six years ago and, in that time, we have NEVER made stuffed peppers. We thought it was high time we right that wrong and give them a bash. Needless to say, you'll be glad we did because these little beauties really are something else. Enjoy!

SERVES 6-8

FOR THE YEMISTA (GREEK STUFFED PEPPERS)
150g basmati rice
12 large mixed peppers
1 large red onion
200g chestnut mushrooms
3 garlic cloves
15g thyme sprigs
4 tbsp extra-virgin olive oil, plus extra for drizzling
2 tsp cumin seeds
2 tsp sea salt
750ml plant-based dry white wine
3 tbsp light soy sauce
600g plant-based mince
2 tsp ground cinnamon
2 tsp dried oregano
2 tsp dried mint
1 vegetable stock cube
220g raisins
4 tbsp tomato purée
100g pine nuts
300ml water
30g fresh dill
20g fresh mint
30g fresh flat-leaf parsley
drizzle of olive oil
sea salt and black pepper

FOR THE EASY TZATZIKI
3 garlic cloves
15g fresh dill
1 cucumber (about 370g)
250g plain plant-based yoghurt (not coconut)
½ lemon
1 tsp sea salt

FOR THE MINTY ROCKET AND KALAMATA SALAD
100g pitted kalamata olives
10g fresh mint
100g rocket
1 lemon

Wok or large frying pan • Frying pan • Roasting tray • Food processor

Prepare the ingredients • Rinse the rice in a sieve under cold running water for 1 minute • Transfer the rice to a bowl, cover with cold water and set to one side • Cut the tops off the peppers and scoop out the seeds and white membranes • Cut a thin slither off the base of the peppers so they're stable when upright • Peel and thinly slice the onion • Cut the mushrooms into olive-sized chunks • Peel and thinly slice the garlic • Pick the thyme leaves

Start cooking the pepper filling • Warm the olive oil in a wok or large frying pan over a high heat • Add the cumin seeds, onion, garlic and 1 teaspoon of salt and fry for 5–6 minutes • Fold in the mushrooms – don't stir too much as you want the mushrooms to caramelise – and cook for 5–10 minutes • Add the wine and soy sauce to deglaze, then reduce the heat and simmer for 10 minutes • Add the mince, cinnamon, thyme, oregano and mint, then crumble in the stock cube and add the raisins, 1 teaspoon of salt and tomato purée and simmer for 15 minutes

Toast the pine nuts • Toast the pine nuts in a dry frying pan over a medium heat for 5 minutes until golden

Finish the filling • Add the toasted pine nuts, drained rice and water to the wok or frying pan, stir and simmer for 12–15 minutes until the rice is tender and all the liquid has been absorbed, stirring occasionally to prevent the rice from catching on the bottom of the wok • Remove from the heat and leave the filling to cool a little bit • Pick the dill fronds and the mint and parsley leaves, roughly chop, add them to the wok and fold into the filling • Preheat oven to 160°C

Build the yemista • Place the peppers in a roasting tray • Spoon the filling into the peppers, making sure they're well stuffed • Top the peppers with their lids, drizzle with a little olive oil, season with salt and pepper and drizzle 3 tablespoons of water into the tray • Put the tray in the oven and roast for 35–40 minutes until the peppers have begun to lightly char on top

Make the tzatziki • Peel and roughly chop the garlic • Pick the dill fronds and roughly chop • Roughly chop the cucumber • Blitz all the ingredients in a food processor, squeezing in the juice from the lemon (catching any pips with your free hand) • Transfer to a bowl

Make the salad • Halve the olives and add them to a bowl • Pick the mint leaves and add them to the bowl with the rocket • Halve the lemon, squeeze over the juice (catching any pips with your free hand) and toss to combine

Time to serve • Transfer the roasted peppers to plates, dress with the salad and serve with the tzatziki (the yemista are also really great served cold)

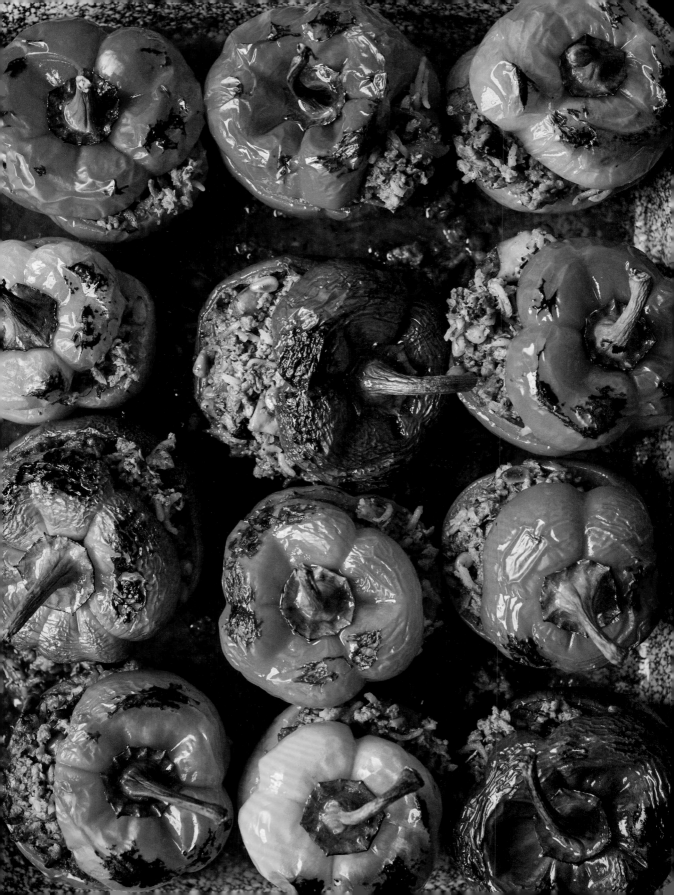

MEATY BHUNA AND AROMATIC PILAU RICE

This is the plant-based curry you wish your local curry house would serve! Thick, dark, delicious gravy with tasty chunks of tofu served over fluffy, flavourful pilau rice. Eaten with your nearest and dearest, this is Friday-night fodder at its finest!

SERVES 4–5

FOR THE LAMB
1 normal breakfast tea bag
1 tsp dried mint
1 tbsp garam masala
2 tbsp light soy sauce
1 litre boiling water
300g soy chunks

FOR THE SPICE MIX
1 tbsp coriander seeds
1 tbsp cumin seeds
1 tbsp fennel seeds
½ tbsp fenugreek seeds
1 tbsp brown mustard seeds

FOR THE CURRY SAUCE
2 onions
5 garlic cloves
2.5cm piece of fresh ginger
1 fresh green chilli
3 tbsp vegetable
    or coconut oil
250ml water
2 x 400g tins chopped
    tomatoes
5 tbsp tomato purée
5cm piece of cinnamon
    stick
1 tbsp garam masala
½ tsp turmeric
1–2 tsp chilli powder
1 tbsp onion powder
1 tbsp light brown sugar
6 cherry tomatoes
1 tbsp white wine vinegar
    or ½ lemon
sea salt

**FOR THE AROMATIC
PILAU RICE**
250g basmati rice
1 onion
1 tbsp vegetable oil
1 tsp cumin seeds
seeds from 2 green
    cardamom pods
2 cloves
1 bay leaf
500ml water
1 tsp plant-based butter

Frying pan • Mortar and pestle or rolling pin • Large saucepan • Medium saucepan • Colander

Prepare the lamb • Put the tea bag, mint, garam masala, soy sauce and boiling water in a large heatproof bowl • Add the soy chunks to the water to rehydrate and cover the bowl to retain the heat • Leave for at least 30 minutes

Make the spice mix • Crush the coriander seeds with a rolling pin or in a mortar and pestle • Heat a dry frying pan over a medium heat, add the cumin seeds, fennel seeds, fenugreek seeds and crushed coriander seeds and toast for a minute until fragrant • Add the mustard seeds and toast for another 1–2 minutes until they start to pop, then remove from the heat and leave to cool a little before transferring to a mortar and pestle and grinding to a powder

Prepare the ingredients for the sauce • Peel and thinly slice the onions and peel and crush the garlic • Peel and finely chop the ginger • Slice the chilli, deseeding it if you want it less spicy

Start making the curry • Heat 2 tablespoons of the vegetable or coconut oil in a large saucepan over a medium heat • Add the onions and cook for about 15 minutes until soft • Add the garlic, ginger and chilli plus a pinch of salt and cook for another 2–3 minutes until the garlic is aromatic • Reduce the heat, add your spice mix and 50ml of the water and simmer for 3–4 minutes • Add the chopped tomatoes, tomato purée, cinnamon stick, a pinch more salt and cover • Simmer over a low heat while you start cooking the rice

Cook the rice • Rinse the rice in a sieve under cold running water for 1 minute • Thinly slice the onion • Heat the vegetable oil in a medium saucepan over a medium heat then add all the dry spices and cook for 1–2 minutes until fragrant • Add the sliced onion and cook for about 10 minutes until it's soft and beginning to go golden • Add the drained rice and stir it through the onion • Pour over the water and bring to the boil then reduce to a simmer • Cover and cook for 12–14 minutes until the water has been absorbed • Turn off the heat, stir through the butter and leave to sit, covered, until ready to serve

While the rice is cooking, finish the curry • Tip the soy chunks into a colander to drain, remove the tea bag and throw it away • Tip the soy chunks and the remaining tablespoon of vegetable oil into the curry and stir to combine • Simmer over a low heat for 15 minutes, add the garam masala and cook for another 7–8 minutes until the soy chunks have doubled in size • Add the turmeric, chilli powder, onion powder, sugar and the remaining 200ml water, then cook for another 10 minutes – the sauce should be thick, deep red and glossy • Halve the cherry tomatoes, add them to the pan and cook for 2–3 more minutes until the tomatoes have softened • Remove from the heat and stir through the white wine vinegar or a squeeze of lemon juice to cut through the spices • Taste and adjust the seasoning (salt/chilli) if required

Time to serve • Serve the curry with the rice on the side • Finish the curry with a swirl of yoghurt, fresh coriander and some crispy fried onions • Garnish the rice with nigella seeds and crispy fried onions

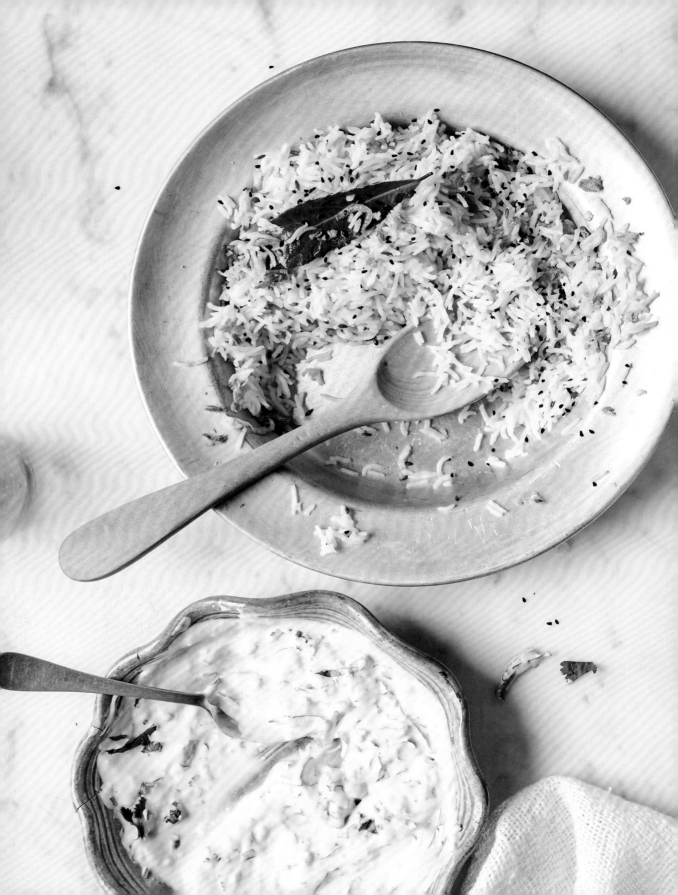

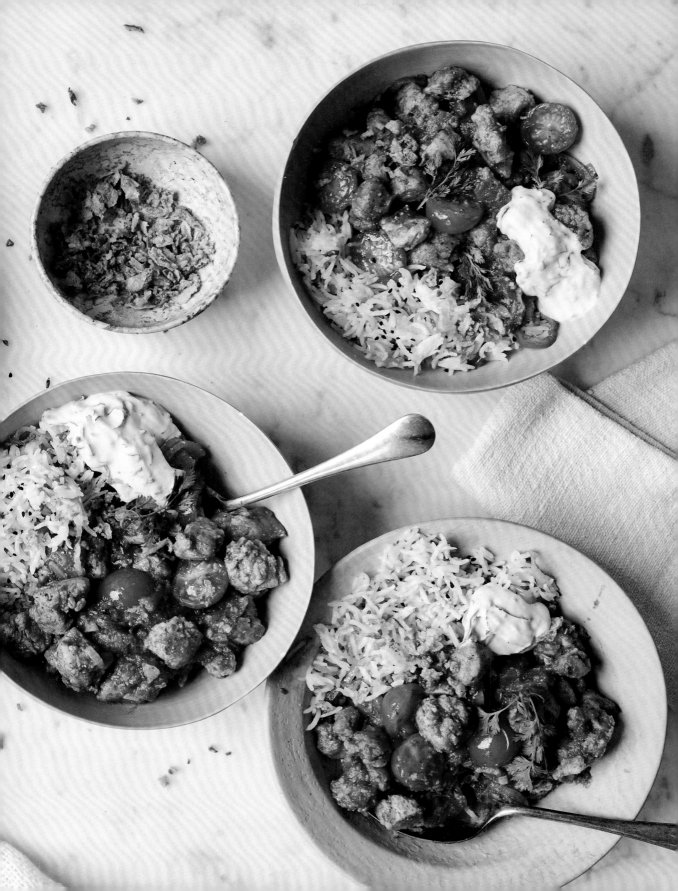

LEBANESE-STYLE LAMB FLATBREADS WITH MINTY YOGHURT

Making flatbread may feel like a labour of love but, really, it involves just a handful of cupboard ingredients and a few kneads to create delicious flatbreads that are impossibly soft on the inside with a glorious golden crust on the outside. You could serve them with anything, but we've stacked them high with a crumbled tempeh lamb spiced with mint, lemon and chilli, and drizzled them with a zesty mint yoghurt. This recipe is good for 2, so if you need to serve 4 simply double everything. Deeeeelicious!

SERVES 2

FOR THE FLATBREADS
140g strong white bread
   flour, plus extra for
   dusting
1 tsp fast-action dried yeast
1 tsp caster sugar
1 tsp baking powder
1 tsp dried mixed herbs
1 tsp table salt
80ml lukewarm water
1 tbsp olive oil
plant-based butter,
   softened, for brushing

FOR THE LAMB TOPPING
300g tempeh
1 onion
2 garlic cloves
splash of olive oil
1 tsp ground cumin
½ tsp ground coriander
½ tsp ground nutmeg
1 tsp smoked paprika
1 tsp chilli powder
2 tbsp mint jelly
1 lemon
sea salt

FOR THE MINT YOGHURT
a few fresh mint leaves
150g plain plant-based
   yoghurt
1 tbsp mint jelly
1 lemon
sea salt

TO SERVE
handful of fresh mint leaves
handful of pomegranate
   seeds
1 tbsp toasted pine nuts
pinch of dried chilli flakes
black pepper

Large saucepan • 2 large flat pans (or 1, and cook the flatbreads in batches) • Pastry brush

Make the flatbread dough • In a large bowl, mix together the dry ingredients (the flour, yeast, sugar, baking powder, mixed herbs and salt) until there are no lumps • Pour in the lukewarm water and olive oil and bring the mixture together to form a dough ball (ensuring you incorporate every part of the mixture) • Place the dough ball on a lightly floured surface and knead for 6–10 minutes until the ball bounces back when pressed • Place the ball back in the bowl, cover and leave somewhere warm for at least 30 minutes

Make the lamb topping • Crumble the tempeh into small pieces using your hands • Peel and dice the onion and garlic • Place a large saucepan over a medium heat and add the olive oil • Add the diced onion, garlic and a pinch of salt • Mix well and cook for 5–10 minutes until the onion begins to soften • At this point, add the spices and crumbled tempeh with a dash of water • Mix well and cook for 5 minutes, then stir through the mint jelly • Halve the lemon and squeeze in some lemon juice, catching any pips in your free hand • Reduce the heat to low and cook for 10 minutes

Make the mint yoghurt • Thinly slice the mint leaves • Put the yoghurt in a small bowl and mix through the mint jelly, sliced mint leaves and a pinch of salt • Halve the lemon and squeeze in some juice, catching any pips in your free hand • Spoon into a small serving bowl

Cook the flatbread • Place 2 large flat pans over a medium heat (over separate flames) • Take the flatbread mixture from the bowl and halve it • Place each piece on a lightly floured work surface and push down using your hands or a rolling pin to create a round, flatbread shape – it should be quite thin as it will become thicker in the pan • Once the pans are hot, add the flatbreads and cook for 2–3 minutes on each side until golden all over and cooked through • If you don't have two flat pans, cook the flatbreads in one flat pan, one at a time

Assemble the flatbreads • Place the flatbreads on 2 serving plates and brush with some butter • Spoon the lamb mixture on top of the flatbreads then drizzle over some mint yoghurt

Time to serve • Chop some mint leaves and sprinkle them over the top of the flatbreads, along with a pinch of black pepper, the pomegranate seeds, pine nuts and chilli flakes (or your favourite toppings)

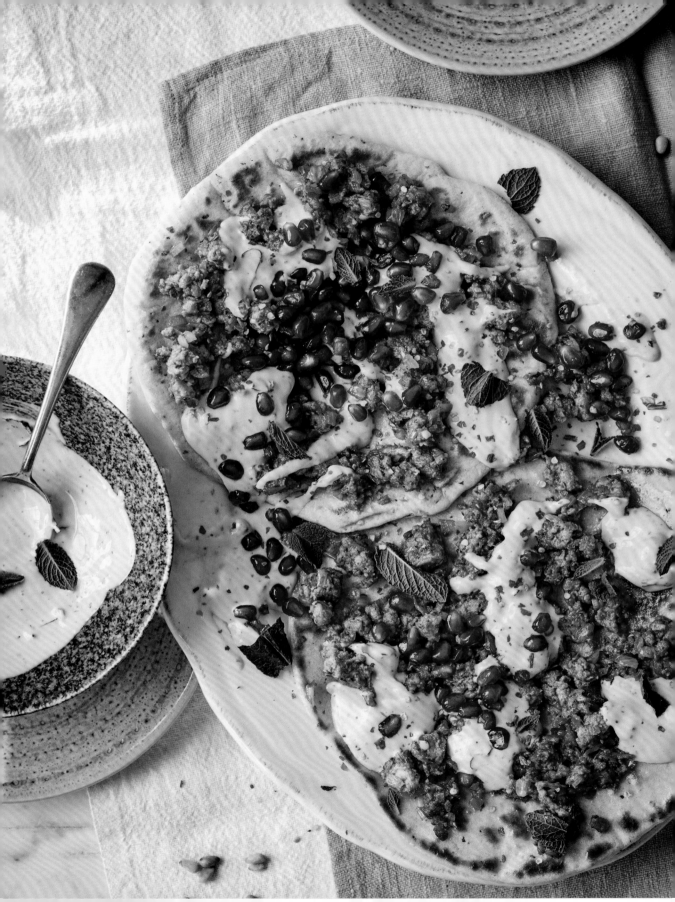

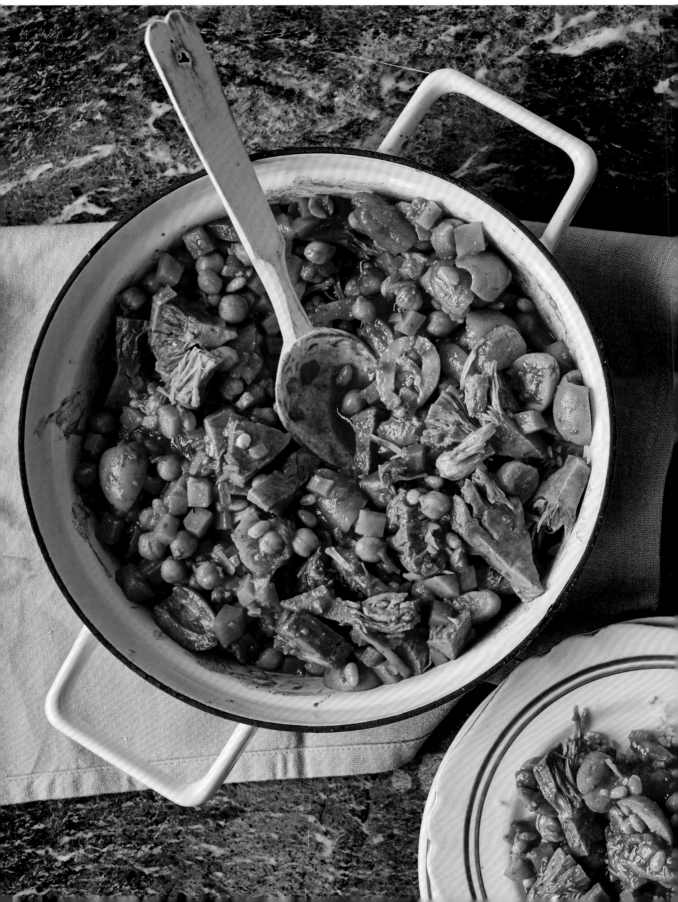

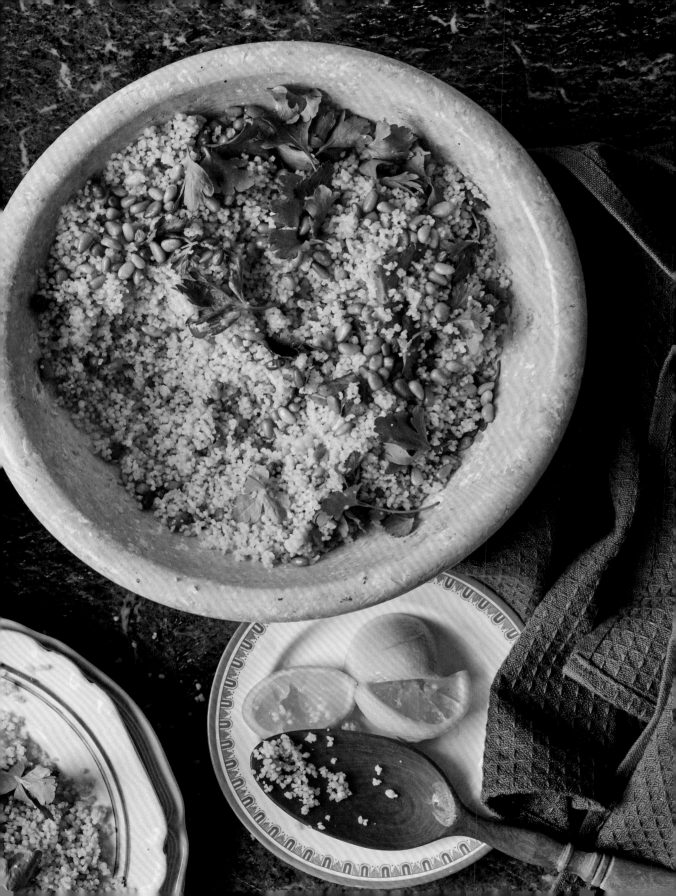

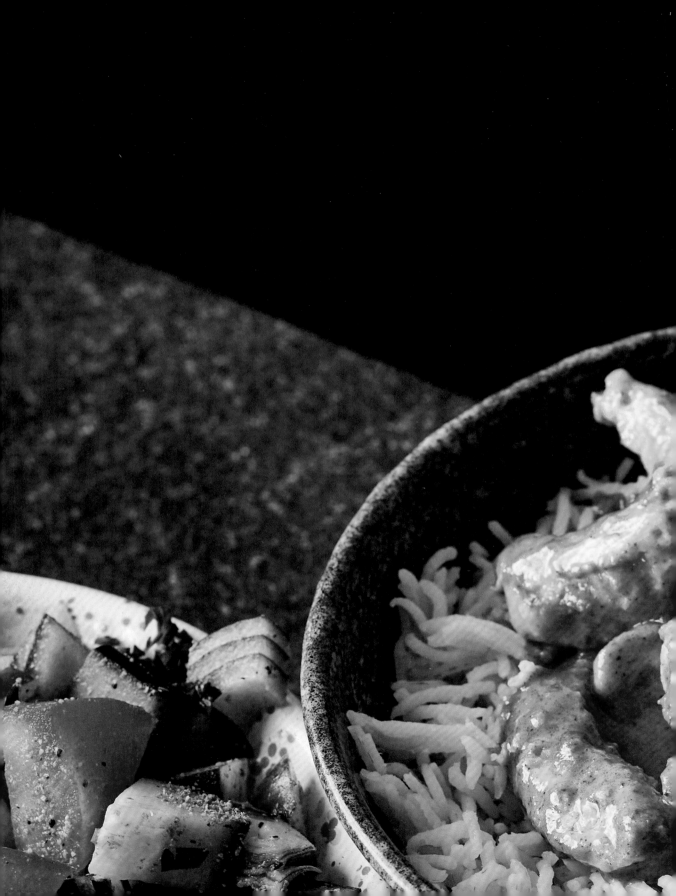

SEAFOOD

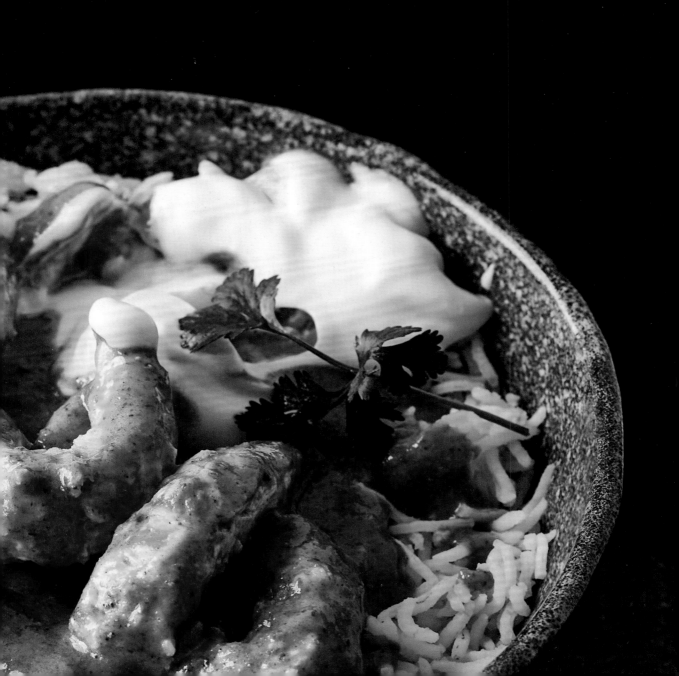

80S PRAWN COCKTAIL

We were both born in the 80s and we both had prawn cocktail for our Christmas dinner starter. In fact, we're pretty sure that more or less everyone who was born in the UK in the 80s had prawn cocktail for their Christmas dinner starter. Pull out the old patterned glassware from the back of the cupboard, make some prawn cocktails and transport yourself back to your childhood. You know you wanna.

SERVES 4–6

**FOR THE MARIE
ROSE SAUCE**
250g plant-based
    mayonnaise
65g ketchup
2 tsp brandy
1 tsp Henderson's relish
½ lemon
1 tsp cayenne pepper, plus
    a little extra to serve
pinch of sea salt
pinch of black pepper

TO SERVE
3 little gem lettuces
2–3 ripe avocados
1 lemon
600g ready-to-eat
    plant-based prawns
    (not breaded)
small bunch of chives
4–6 slices of brown bread
plant-based butter, for
    spreading

Whisk • Glasses to serve in

Make the marie rose sauce • Put all the ingredients in a bowl, squeezing in the juice from the half lemon (catching any pips in your free hand) and whisk together to form a lovely creamy sauce • Check the seasoning and adjust if needed

Prepare the salad ingredients • Pick and wash the gem lettuce leaves, pat the leaves dry and reserve 3 nice leaves per serving • Thinly slice the remaining leaves • Remove the stones from the avocados, peel off the skin and slice each avocado half into 6 wedges • Cut the lemon into neat wedges, removing the pips if needed

Prepare the prawn cocktails • Divide the sliced gem lettuce among the serving glasses • Mix the prawns in half the marie rose sauce • Place a portion of prawns on each bed of gem lettuce • Garnish with a wedge of lemon, 5 slices of avocado, the reserved gem leaves and a lovely big spoon of the remaining marie rose sauce

Time to serve • Chop the chives • Spread the brown bread with butter, sprinkle a little cayenne and chopped chives over the marie rose and serve immediately, alongside the bread

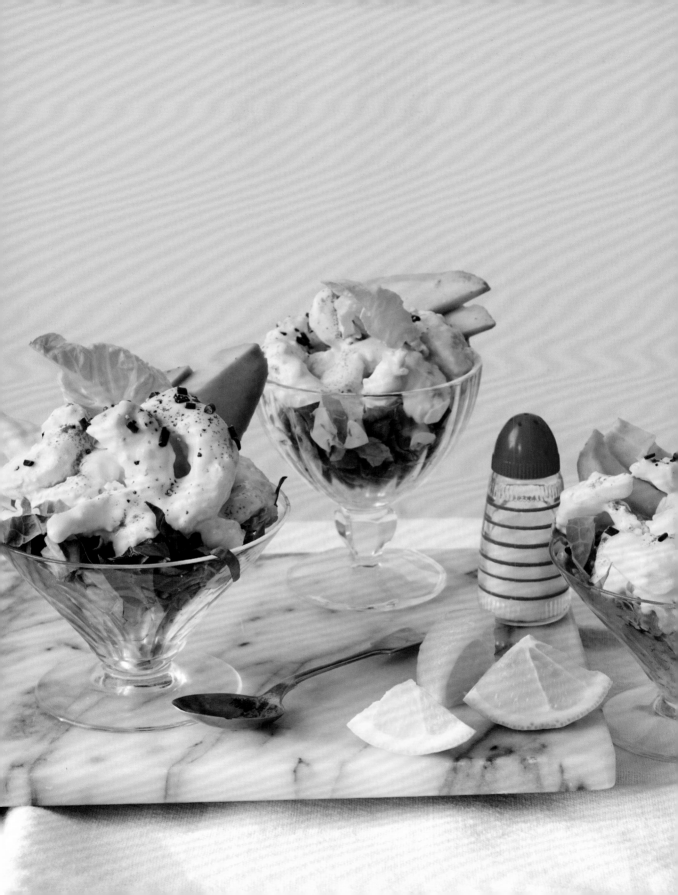

FILLET – WOAH – FISH

Fillet that makes you say 'WOAH'. Sauce that makes you say 'WOAH'. Fries that make you say 'WOAH'. A meal that'll make you and all your mates say 'WOAH'. Fair to say you WOAH-n't be disappointed with this one. Cheers Ronald, we'll take it from here.

SERVES 4

**FOR THE FILLET
– WOAH – FISH**
400g extra-firm tofu
2 nori sheets
2 tbsp brine from a jar
    of capers
2 tbsp brine from a jar
    of gherkins
½ lemon
4 tbsp egg replacement
8 tbsp water
80g plain flour
300g plain breadcrumbs
sea salt and black pepper

FOR THE FRIES
4 large Maris Piper potatoes
vegetable oil, for deep-
    shallow frying
sea salt

**FOR THE TARTARE
SAUCE**
1 small shallot
3 tbsp capers in vinegar
3 tbsp gherkins
15g fresh flat-leaf parsley
1 lemon
120g plant-based
    mayonnaise
sea salt, black pepper
    and sugar

TO FINISH
4 plant-based brioche buns
drizzle of olive oil
4 slices of plant-based
    cheese

Scissors • 2 large saucepans • Pastry brush • 2 baking trays • Frying pan • Probe thermometer • Metal slotted spoon

Prepare the tofu • Drain and pat dry the tofu with kitchen paper, then cut it into 4 equal slices • Use scissors to cut one of the sheets of nori into pieces • Place the nori pieces in a wide, shallow bowl and add the caper brine, gherkin brine and a little salt and pepper • Squeeze the lemon juice into the bowl, catching any pips in your free hand • Stir to combine • Lay the tofu slices in the bowl and leave to marinate, turning them a couple of times to coat them in the marinade

Prepare the fries • Peel the potatoes and cut into fries • Rinse the fries in a few changes of cold water to wash off the starch, place in a large saucepan and cover with cold water • Season with a good pinch of salt and bring to the boil over a high heat • When the water starts to bubble, set a timer for 5 minutes • Drain the fries and allow to steam-dry until cold • Preheat oven to 150°C

Make the Fillet – WOAH – Fish • Stir the egg replacement and water together in a shallow bowl, adding more water if necessary • Quarter the remaining nori sheet • Remove the marinated tofu from the bowl, lay on a clean surface, place the quartered nori on top of the tofu and rest for a minute (so the nori sticks to the tofu) • Put the flour in a shallow bowl, place the tofu slices in the bowl and use a teaspoon to cover and coat the tofu • Brush the tofu slices all over with egg replacement, cover with breadcrumbs and repeat so the tofu is double-breaded for extra crunch • Place on a baking tray ready to fry

Make the tartare sauce • Peel and finely dice the shallot • Drain and roughly chop the capers • Dice the gherkins • Pick the parsley leaves and finely chop • Halve the lemon and squeeze the juice into a bowl • Add the shallots, capers, gherkins, parsley, mayo, and a little salt, pepper and sugar, and stir to combine

Prepare the buns • Halve the buns and drizzle with a little oil • Toast in a dry frying pan over a medium-high heat, cut side down, for a minute or two until golden

Cook the fries and fillets • Warm the oil in a large saucepan to 180°C (use a thermometer) • Use a metal slotted spoon to lower the fries into the oil and fry for 5–6 minutes until golden and crispy (you may have to do this in batches) • Drain the fries, spread them out on a baking tray, season and place the tray in the oven to keep the fries warm and crispy • Once the fries are cooked, fry the fillets in the oil for 4–5 minutes until golden and crispy • Remove the fillets from the pan and place on a plate lined with kitchen paper to soak up any excess oil

Time to serve • Lay the plant-based cheese on the bottom halves of the toasted buns, top with the fillets, dress with the tartare sauce, top with the top halves of the toasted buns and serve immediately with the fries

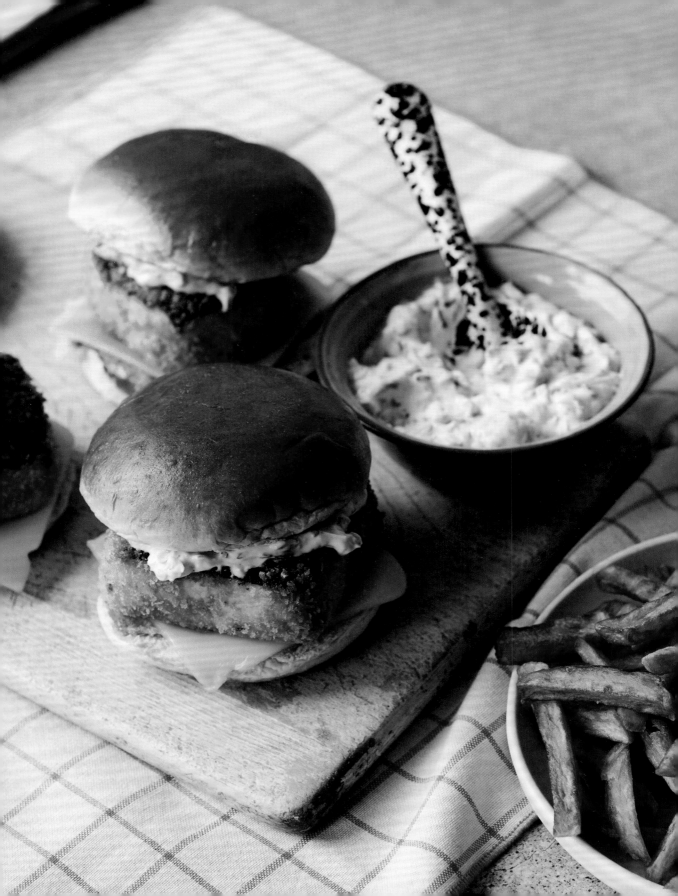

DATE-NIGHT SCALLOPS

Sarah and Ian went on holiday to Lisbon in May 2022 and fell in love with the place. Great vibes, lovely people, interesting history, marvellous weather, fantastic architecture but – most importantly – phenomenal food. They visited a restaurant called Ao 26 that served delicious plant-based scallops, which inspired them to include this recipe in the book. Hope you enjoy them!

SERVES 2

FOR THE SCALLOPS
3 fat king oyster mushrooms
1 tbsp vegetable oil
1 tbsp plant-based butter
½ lemon
sea salt and black pepper

FOR THE ASPARAGUS
300g thick asparagus spears

FOR THE SEAWEED BUTTER
2 garlic cloves
75g plant-based butter
1 tbsp nori or dulse seaweed flakes

FOR THE HAZELNUTS
50g hazelnuts
1 tbsp linseeds
1 tbsp sunflower seeds
1 tsp rapeseed oil

Preheat oven to 200°C • Medium saucepan • Baking tray • Ovenproof frying pan

Prepare the mushroom scallops • Cut the caps and the uneven bases away from the mushrooms and save for another recipe • Cut the stems of the mushrooms into 2.5cm-thick slices (these are the scallops) • Use a sharp knife to lightly score both sides of the mushroom slices in a criss-cross pattern

Prepare the asparagus • Snap off and discard the woody ends of the asparagus spears then peel the bases • Slice in half on an angle • Set aside

Make the seaweed butter • Finely chop the garlic • Melt the butter in a medium saucepan over a medium heat, add the seaweed flakes and let the garlic and seaweed infuse the butter • Remove from the heat, place the trimmed and sliced asparagus in the pan and toss in the butter

Toast the hazelnuts • Spread out the hazelnuts and seeds on a baking tray, drizzle with the oil and roast in the oven for 4–5 minutes • Remove the tray from the oven, tip the nuts and seeds onto a chopping board, leave to cool for a couple of minutes, then roughly chop the nuts

Cook the mushroom scallops • Warm the vegetable oil in an ovenproof frying pan over a medium-high heat • Place all the scallops into the pan and fry for 2–3 minutes until they're turning golden • Flip the scallops over, add the butter and season with a little salt and pepper • Place the pan in the oven and roast for 5 minutes

Time to serve • Halve the half lemon into wedges for the scallops • Quickly cook the asparagus in the seaweed butter for about 2 minutes • Plate the asparagus and scallops, dress with the seaweed butter, sprinkle over the nuts and seeds and serve immediately with the lemon wedges

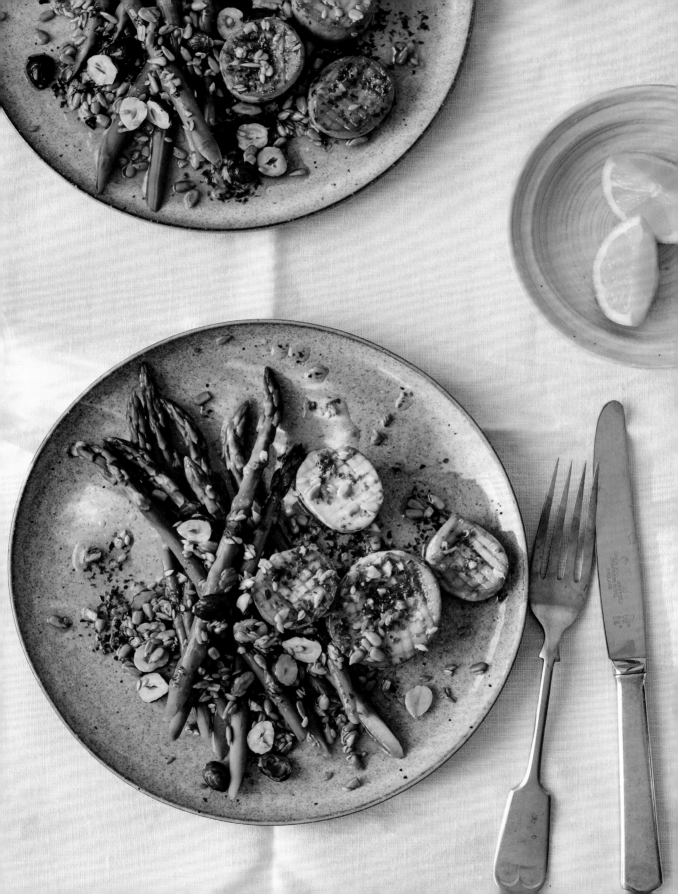

MOQUECA (BRAZILIAN FISH STEW)

This Brazilian stew is fully loaded with beautiful, bright flavours that will make you want to go on holiday. Serve it with rice, kinda like a curry, or serve it in a bowl, kinda like a soup. Either way, Moqueca is sunshine in a pot.

SERVES 4

FOR THE RICE
½ white onion
1 garlic clove
1 tbsp extra-virgin olive oil
210g long-grain white rice
500ml boiling water
pinch of sea salt

FOR THE STEW
1 red onion
2 carrots
1 red pepper
1 yellow pepper
3 garlic cloves
½ fresh jalapeño chilli
400g fresh tomatoes
3 tbsp coconut oil
½ tsp salt
1 tbsp tomato purée
2 tsp paprika
1 tsp ground cumin
1 x 400g tin banana blossom
150g plant-based prawns
1 x 400g tin coconut milk
250ml vegetable stock
2 limes
sea salt and black pepper

TO SERVE
10g fresh coriander
1 lime

Fine grater or microplane • Medium saucepan • Large saucepan

Cook the rice • Peel and dice the onion • Peel and grate the garlic • Warm the olive oil in a medium saucepan, add the onion and salt, then fry for 3–4 minutes until softened • Add the garlic and fry for a further minute • Rinse the rice in a sieve under cold running water for 1 minute • Add the rice and boiling water to the pan, set the heat to medium, put the lid on, slightly ajar, and simmer for 15 minutes • Take the pan off the heat, close the lid fully and leave to steam

Prepare the vegetables for the moqueca • Peel and finely dice the onion and carrots • Halve, core and dice the peppers • Peel and grate the garlic • Halve, deseed and dice the jalapeño • Dice the tomatoes

Start making the moqueca • Warm the coconut oil in the large saucepan over a medium heat • Add all the diced and grated ingredients and the salt and cook, stirring, for 7–8 minutes to soften • Add the tomato purée, paprika and cumin and stir for 2 minutes • Add the tomatoes to the pan and cook for 8–10 minutes, stirring occasionally to prevent the mixture catching on the bottom of the pan

Finish the moqueca • Rinse the tinned banana blossom under cold water to wash off the brine and roughly chop it into bite-sized pieces • Put the banana blossom and the prawns in the saucepan and pour over the coconut milk and vegetable stock • Reduce the heat so the moqueca is simmering gently and cook for 13–15 minutes

Time to serve • Halve the 2 limes and squeeze the juice (you should have about 4 tablespoons) into the pan • Taste the sauce and season to perfection with salt and pepper • Pick the coriander leaves and sprinkle over the moqueca • Fluff up the rice with a fork and spoon into bowls, top with the moqueca and serve immediately with a third lime cut into wedges

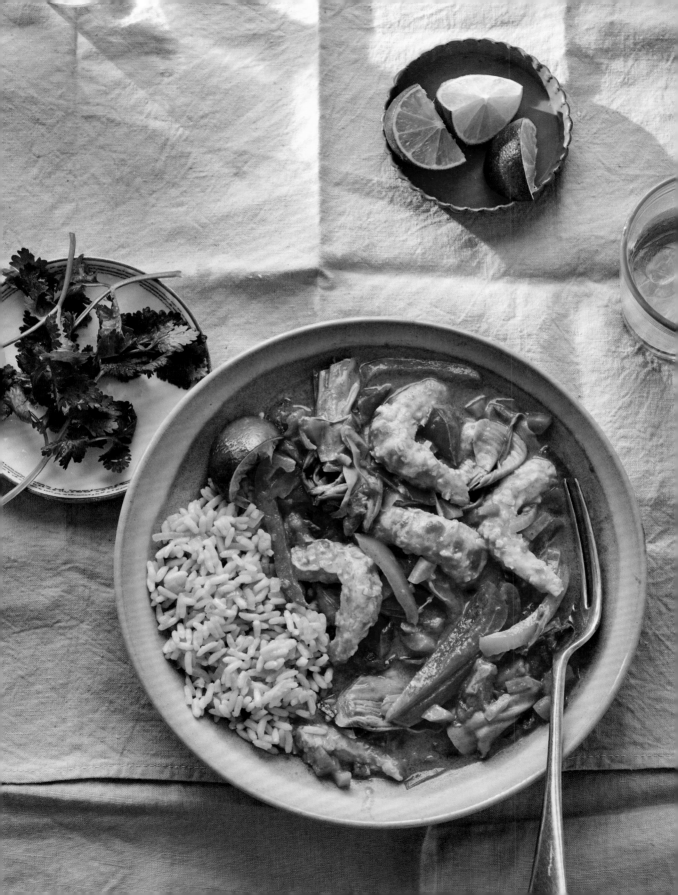

BAKED TUNA PUTTANESCA WITH CRISPY GNOCCHI

This technique for cooking gnocchi is like knowing a magic trick. Seriously, it's like creating gold nuggets from lumps of dough. You'll come back to it time and time again. As for the sauce, well, where do we start? It's rich beyond comprehension, and you'll dream of the flavours for weeks afterwards. It's made from cooking down onion and garlic before mixing through plant-based tuna, capers, black olives and tomatoes and leaving it to simmer to perfection. We pile it on top of the crispy gnocchi for a match made in heaven and a meal you quite simply have to try.

SERVES 4

FOR THE TUNA PUTTANESCA SAUCE
1 onion
2 garlic cloves
drizzle of olive oil
1 vegetable stock cube
200ml boiling water
2 tbsp capers in vinegar
75g good-quality pitted black olives
150g plant-based tuna
1 tsp dried chilli flakes (add more if you like it spicy)
1 x 400g tin good-quality chopped tomatoes
1 tbsp rose harissa paste
1 tbsp thick balsamic vinegar
1 tbsp light brown sugar
2 tbsp nooch (nutritional yeast), plus extra for sprinkling
sea salt and black pepper

FOR THE GNOCCHI
500g potato gnocchi
3 garlic cloves
2 tbsp olive oil
2 tbsp plant-based butter
2 tbsp nooch (nutritional yeast)
sea salt and black pepper

TO SERVE
handful of fresh basil leaves
toasted pine nuts

Preheat oven to 180°C • Shallow casserole dish • Kettle boiled • Non-stick saucepan

Make the puttanesca sauce • Peel and very finely dice the onion and garlic • Place a shallow casserole dish over a medium heat and add the olive oil • Once warm, add the diced onion, garlic and a pinch of salt • Mix well and cook for 5–10 minutes, or until the onion softens • Mix the stock cube and boiling water until dissolved • Drain and finely chop the capers and olives and add them to the onion and garlic in the pan • Add the tuna and break it up using a wooden spoon • Mix through the chilli flakes and cook for 1 minute • Add the chopped tomatoes, harissa paste, stock, balsamic vinegar and sugar and stir to combine • Bring to the boil, then place the pan in the oven and roast the sauce as you cook and then fry the gnocchi (the sauce will be happy in the oven for anything from 15 to 30 minutes)

Cook the gnocchi • Add the gnocchi to a non-stick saucepan of boiling water and cook according to the packet instructions (or until the gnocchi rises to the surface) • Once cooked, drain the gnocchi in a colander and set to one side

Fry the gnocchi • Peel and very roughly chop the garlic • Place the dry gnocchi pan back over a high heat and add the olive oil and butter • Once the butter has melted, add the chopped garlic and cook for a couple of minutes to infuse the flavour before removing the garlic • Add the drained gnocchi and mix through • Fry the gnocchi until golden and crispy on all sides, stirring constantly • Once the gnocchi is golden and crispy, drain off the excess oil – this can be done by tipping the frying pan slightly and spooning out the oil • Mix through the nooch and a little salt and pepper • Toss everything together to combine

Finish the dish • Thinly slice the basil leaves • Remove the pan of sauce from the oven and season with salt and pepper • Stir through the chopped basil (saving some for the top), nooch and two-thirds of the gnocchi – if the sauce is too thick, you can mix through a dash of water

Time to serve • Spoon the sauce into serving bowls and add the remaining gnocchi on top • Dress the dishes with more chopped basil, pine nuts, nooch and ground pepper • Serve immediately

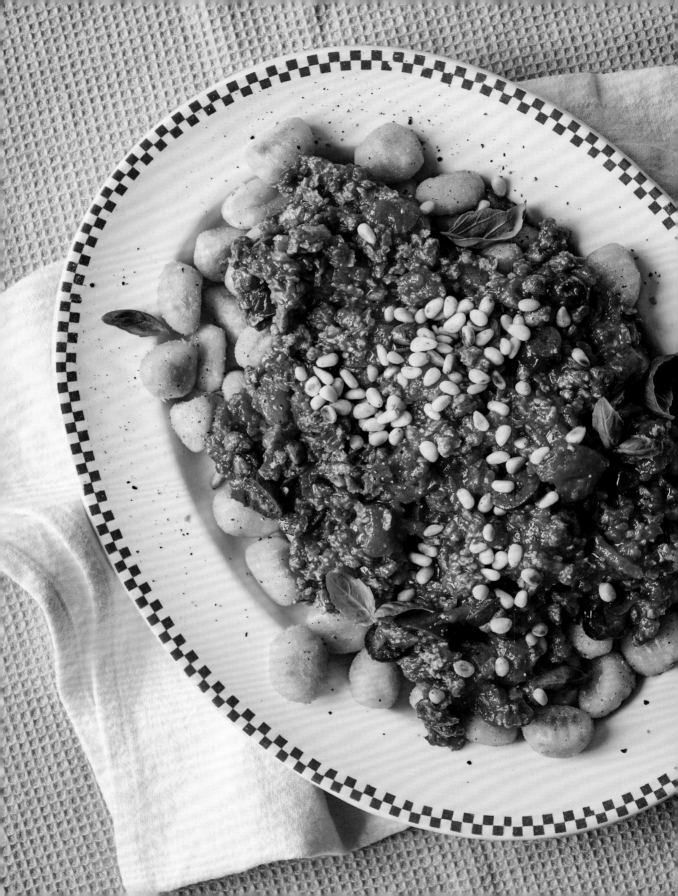

CHOW-DOWN CHOWDER

Smooth soup is great but when you have a soup with texture, the game changes. A little crunch here, a little crisp there, this is a recipe that has the potential to really knock your socks off. If you enjoy creamy, buttery, silky sensations and appreciate a little smoke, you've just hit the jackpot.

**SERVES 2 AS A MAIN,
4 AS A SMALL STARTER**

1 onion
3 celery sticks
25g plant-based butter
2 tbsp plain flour
500ml vegetable stock
500ml unsweetened
    soy milk
200g new potatoes
200g firm smoked tofu
120g button mushrooms
200g frozen sweetcorn
3 tbsp nori sprinkles (or
    more, to taste)
drizzle of olive oil
a few drops of liquid smoke,
    to taste (optional)
smoked sea salt and
    black pepper

TO SERVE
2 spring onions
small bunch of fresh
    flat-leaf parsley
1 lemon

Large saucepan • Measuring jug • Frying pan

Prepare and cook the vegetables • Peel and dice the onion • Trim and dice the celery, removing any fibrous strands • Warm the butter in a large saucepan over a medium heat, add the onion and celery and sweat for about 7 minutes until soft • Add the plain flour and stir for 1–2 minutes

Make the broth • Gradually add the stock and milk to the pan, whisking to avoid the mixture clumping • Bring the soup to a simmer • While the soup is simmering, peel and quarter the potatoes and add them to the soup (you can keep the skin on if you prefer) • Cook the soup with the potatoes for 15–17 minutes until the potatoes are tender

Prepare the tofu and mushrooms • Tip any water from the tofu pack into the soup and rip the block into small shreds • Trim the mushroom stalks and cut the stalks in half • Add the tofu, sweetcorn, nori sprinkles and a good pinch of pepper to the pan and simmer for 5 minutes • While the soup is simmering, heat the olive oil in a frying pan over a medium heat, add the mushrooms and fry for 5 minutes • Taste and add a little liquid smoke to taste (if using)

Time to serve • Add the mushrooms to the pan and stir into the soup • Taste and season with smoked salt • Trim and thinly slice the spring onions • Pick and chop the parsley leaves • Quarter the lemon • Ladle the soup into bowls, garnish with spring onions and parsley and serve immediately with a lemon quarter for squeezing

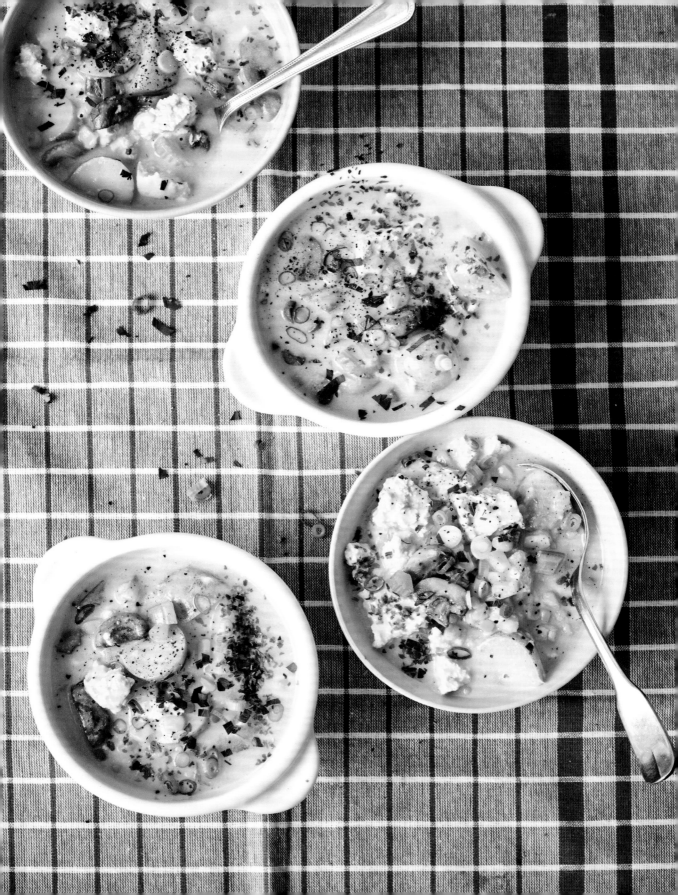

LOBSTER ROLL

Imagine a prawn sandwich with superpowers; that's what this is. Thick, velvety sauce, deliciously meaty lobster and crispy, crunchy lettuce all wrapped up in a golden brioche bun. It sounds good, it looks good and trust us, it is really, really good.

SERVES 4

FOR THE LOBSTER
1 lemon
1 tbsp Cajun spice mix
2 tbsp olive oil
2 x 410g tins hearts of palm
sea salt and black pepper

FOR THE SAUCE
1 lemon
1 celery stalk
2 echalion shallots
3 dill sprigs
90g plant-based
    mayonnaise
1 tsp nori sprinkles
pinch of sea salt

TO SERVE
4 plant-based brioche
    hot dog rolls
plant-based butter,
    for spreading
1 baby gem lettuce
black pepper

Frying pan

Prepare the hearts of palm • Cut the lemon in half and squeeze the juice into a mixing bowl, catching any pips in your free hand • Add the Cajun spice, 1 tablespoon of the olive oil and a pinch each of salt and pepper and stir to combine • Drain the hearts of palm and rinse under cold running water • Lay out on a chopping board and roughly chop • Add the hearts of palm to the mixing bowl and stir gently to coat • Heat the remaining olive oil in a frying pan over a medium heat • Once warm, add the marinated hearts of palm to the pan and fry for 5 minutes until starting to char on the sides • Once cooked, transfer the hearts of palm to a bowl and set to one side to cool

Make the sauce • Halve the lemon and squeeze the juice of one half into a mixing bowl, catching any pips in your free hand • Trim and very finely dice the celery • Peel, trim and very finely dice the shallots • Remove the fronds from the dill sprigs and chop finely • Add the mayo, chopped celery, shallots, dill, nori sprinkles and salt to the mixing bowl and mix well until everything comes together

Combine the elements • Add the sauce to the bowl of hearts of palm and mix well to combine • Place the bowl in the fridge to chill

Prepare the rest of the ingredients • Cut the hot dog rolls in half and toast • Once toasted, butter every side of each role • Cut the ends of the lettuce and shred

Build the sandwiches • Load up the rolls with the lettuce and filling • Sprinkle with a little black pepper and serve immediately

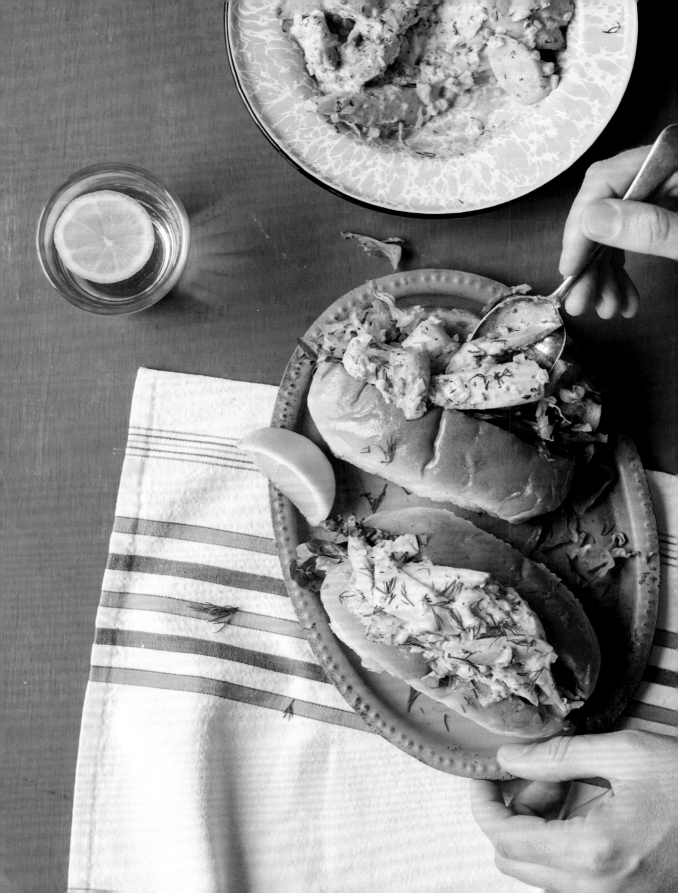

TUSCAN TUNA PASTA SALAD

There's a very high chance this dish will find its way into your weekly recipe repertoire because it's simple, it's easy and it's extremely delicious. When we make this, we tend to make a biggish batch as it's perfect for a pack-up lunch the next day, and great with a dollop of hummus too. This kinda goes without saying but the better the olive, the better the flavour; we like those big fat ones you get at posh food markets.

SERVES 4

2 litres water
large pinch of sea salt
300g dried short pasta
    (elbow macaroni
    or radiatore)
1 red onion
12 good-quality large green
    olives
240g baby plum tomatoes
1 celery stick
1 x 400g tin borlotti beans
150g plant-based tuna
good-quality extra-virgin
    olive oil
30g fresh flat-leaf parsley
½ lemon
sea salt and black pepper

Kettle boiled • Large saucepan

Cook the pasta • Get the 2 litres of water bubbling a large saucepan over a high heat and sprinkle in the salt • Add the pasta to the pan and cook according to the packet instructions for al dente (about 8–9 minutes), then drain in a colander and set aside

Prepare the salad ingredients • Peel and thinly slice the red onion and soak it in cold water • Halve, destone and thickly slice the olives • Quarter the baby plum tomatoes • Trim and thinly slice the celery • Rinse and drain the borlotti beans

Build the salad • Drain the onion and add it to a salad bowl • Add the beans, tomatoes, olives and celery and toss to combine • Flake the tuna into the bowl along with a good glug of extra-virgin olive oil and the pasta and gently fold to combine • Pick the parsley leaves and finely chop (saving a few leaves for garnish) • Squeeze the lemon juice into the bowl, catching any pips in your free hand • Sprinkle in the parsley and fold to combine • Taste and season to perfection with salt and pepper

Time to serve • Spoon the salad into bowls, garnish with parsley and serve immediately

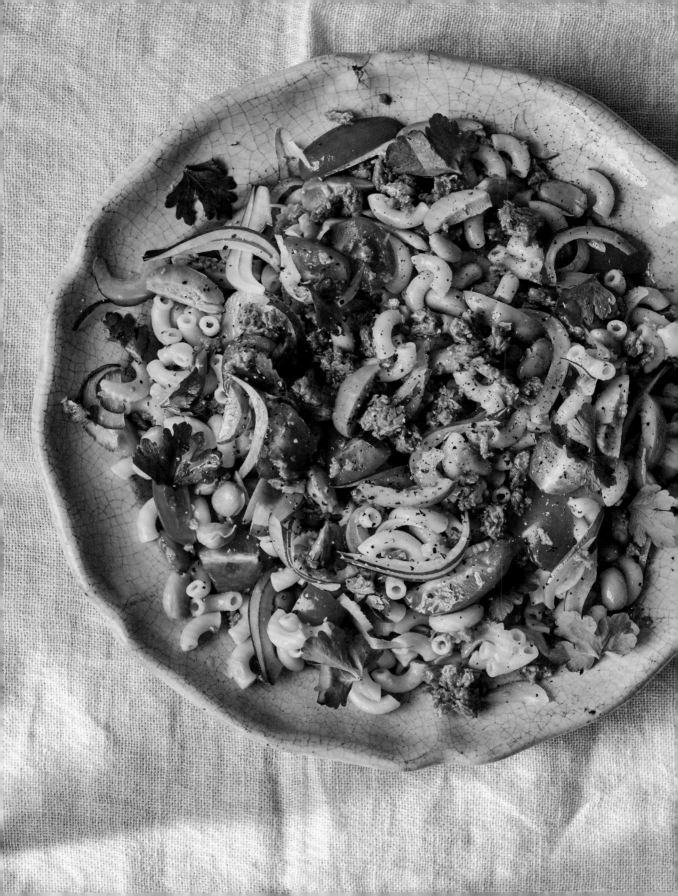

PRAWN MALAI

If you've followed us for a while, you'll be well aware we love a curry. We've done bhunas, kormas, jalfrezis, madrases, rogan joshes but we've never tackled a malai. Because of that, we thought it was high time to give this Bengali classic the BOSH! treatment. It has lovely flavours, great creamy texture and looks fantastic. An all-round tip-top curry that we're sure you'll love as much as we do!

SERVES 4

FOR THE PRAWNS
400g plant-based prawns
2 tbsp vegetable oil
1 tsp turmeric
1 tsp garlic powder
1 tsp sea salt

FOR THE CURRY PASTE
2 onions
6 garlic cloves
2.5cm piece of fresh ginger
4 green cardamom pods
2 bay leaves
5cm piece of cinnamon stick
2 cloves or ½ tsp ground cloves
1 fresh green chilli
drop of neutral oil

FOR THE RICE
300g basmati rice
600ml cold water
½ tsp fine sea salt

FOR THE CURRY SAUCE
2 tbsp vegetable oil
2 tbsp garam masala
2 tsp red chilli powder
1 tsp turmeric
2 tsp ground cinnamon
2 tbsp light brown sugar
1 x 400g tin coconut milk
100g plant-based yoghurt
100ml water
2 tbsp plant-based
   ghee or butter

FOR THE KACHUMBER
2 tomatoes
½ cucumber
½ red onion
2 sprigs of coriander
2 sprigs of mint
½ tsp ground black pepper
½ tsp ground cumin
½ tsp ground coriander
½ lemon

TO SERVE (OPTIONAL)
plant-based double cream
fresh coriander

Defrost the prawns if frozen • Frying pan • Powerful blender • Medium saucepan

Prepare the prawns • Mix the oil, turmeric, garlic powder and salt together in a bowl • Toss the prawns in the mixture and set aside

Make the curry paste • Peel and quarter the onions and peel the garlic and ginger • Remove the seeds from the cardamom pods • Heat a dry frying pan over a medium heat, add the whole spices and cook for 2 minutes until fragrant, stirring them frequently so they don't burn • Transfer the spices to a powerful blender and blitz to a powder • Add the onion, garlic, ginger, chilli and oil to the blender and blitz to a paste, adding a splash of water to help bring the paste together if needed

Cook the rice • Rinse the rice in a sieve under cold running water for 1 minute • Tip into a saucepan, pour over the water and add the salt • Cover the pan and bring to the boil over a high heat • When the water starts to boil, turn down the heat to low and cook covered for 12 minutes • Take the pan off the heat, keep the lid on and leave to steam

Make the curry sauce • In the same pan you toasted the spices in, heat the vegetable oil over a medium heat • Add the curry paste and cook for about 5 minutes until soft, fragrant and golden • Add the prawns and cook for 2–3 minutes to sear them and infuse them with flavours (or cook for however long it states on the packet) then remove from pan and set aside • Stir through the garam masala, chilli powder, turmeric, cinnamon and sugar, then pour in the coconut milk, yoghurt and water and stir to combine • Add salt to taste, reduce the heat and cook for 5–7 minutes until the sauce has thickened • Add the ghee or butter at the end and stir through – it should be rich and creamy, with the oil slightly separating from the cream • Stir through the cooked prawns and remove from the heat

Make the kachumber • Dice the tomato, cucumber and red onion into even-sized pieces – your choice of chunkiness • Finely chop the coriander and mint • Mix together in a bowl and season with salt, then add the pepper, cumin, coriander and squeeze the lemon juice through, catching any pips in your free hand

Time to serve • Spoon the rice and prawn malai into a bowl (warming the prawns and sauce through first, for a couple of minutes, if needed), dress with kachumba and swirl over a little plant-based cream (if using) • Chop the coriander, sprinkle it on top and serve immediately

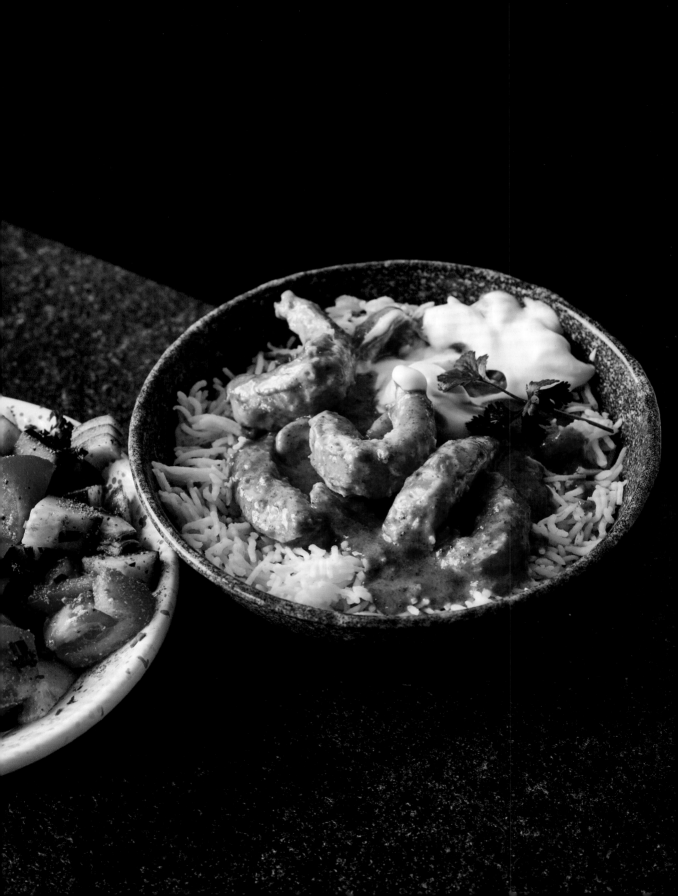

BACON FISHCAKES WITH MINTY PEA MASH AND LEMON HOLLANDAISE SAUCE

If you've got people coming round for dinner and you want to make them something a bit special, this could be what you're looking for. It looks great, it tastes great, it's quite hearty but not too heavy and pairs really well with a good glass of white wine. Posh gastro pub food at home – sounds like a win to us!

SERVES 4

FOR THE LEMON HOLLANDAISE SAUCE
200g raw unsalted cashews
300ml boiling water
1½ lemons
2 tbsp nooch (nutritional yeast)
½ ground turmeric
½ tsp sea salt
½ Dijon mustard

FOR THE BACON FISHCAKES
300g Charlotte potatoes
1 tsp sea salt
2 strips of plant-based bacon
6 spring onions
10g fresh chives
20g fresh flat-leaf parsley
2 lemons
3 tbsp Henderson's relish
4 tbsp panko breadcrumbs, plus extra for rolling
300g plant-based tuna
120g plant-based cream
3 tbsp vegetable oil

FOR THE MINTY PEA MASH
3 garlic cloves
2 echalion shallots
2 tbsp vegetable oil
100ml boiling water
250g frozen peas
250g frozen broad beans
10g fresh mint leaves
6 tbsp plant-based cream
½ tsp sea salt

TO SERVE
handful of fresh chives
large handful of watercress
squeeze of lemon juice

2 saucepans • Box grater • Large frying pan • Powerful blender

Prepare the cashews for the sauce • Put the cashews in a heatproof bowl and cover with boiling water • Set aside for 30 minutes to hydrate and soften

Cook the potatoes • Halve the potatoes, put them in a saucepan with the salt, cover with water, place over a high heat and bring to the boil, then reduce the heat and simmer for 18–20 minutes until soft • Drain the potatoes and leave to cool for a few minutes before crushing with a fork

Prepare the other fishcake ingredients • Dice the bacon • Trim and thinly slice the spring onions and finely chop the chives • Pick the parsley leaves and thinly slice • Zest the lemons with the fine side of a box grater

Build the fishcakes • Add the bacon, spring onions, parsley leaves, lemon zest, Henderson's relish and breadcrumbs to the bowl of potatoes, flake in the tuna and stir to combine • Slowly drizzle the cream into the bowl while folding into the mixture • Form into 12 cakes with neat sides and flat tops and chill for about 30 minutes in the fridge until firm

Make the minty pea mash • Peel and finely dice the garlic and shallots • Heat the oil in a saucepan over a medium heat, add the garlic and shallots and sauté for 3–5 minutes until soft • Add the boiling water, frozen peas and broad beans and simmer for 2 minutes • Remove from the heat and leave to cool for a couple of minutes • Add the contents of the pan, mint, cream and salt to the blender and pulse to combine • The texture should be chopped and have bite, not be puréed • Transfer to a bowl and clean out the blender

Make the sauce • Squeeze the lemon juice into the blender (catching any pips in your free hand), add the cashews (and a little of the soaking water) along with the nooch, turmeric, salt and Dijon mustard • Blend until completely smooth, adding more soaking water if necessary

Finish the fishcakes • Remove the fishcakes from the fridge and roll each one evenly in breadcrumbs, making sure they're well covered • Heat the vegetable oil in a frying pan over a medium heat • Carefully lay the fishcakes in the pan and fry for about 4 minutes on each side until golden and crispy (if you have a large enough frying pan, cook all the fishcakes in one go, otherwise fry them in batches)

Time to serve • Finely chop the chives • Spoon the mash on to plates • Top with 3 fishcakes each, dress with watercress, garnish with chives, finish with a little lemon juice and serve immediately with the sauce on the side

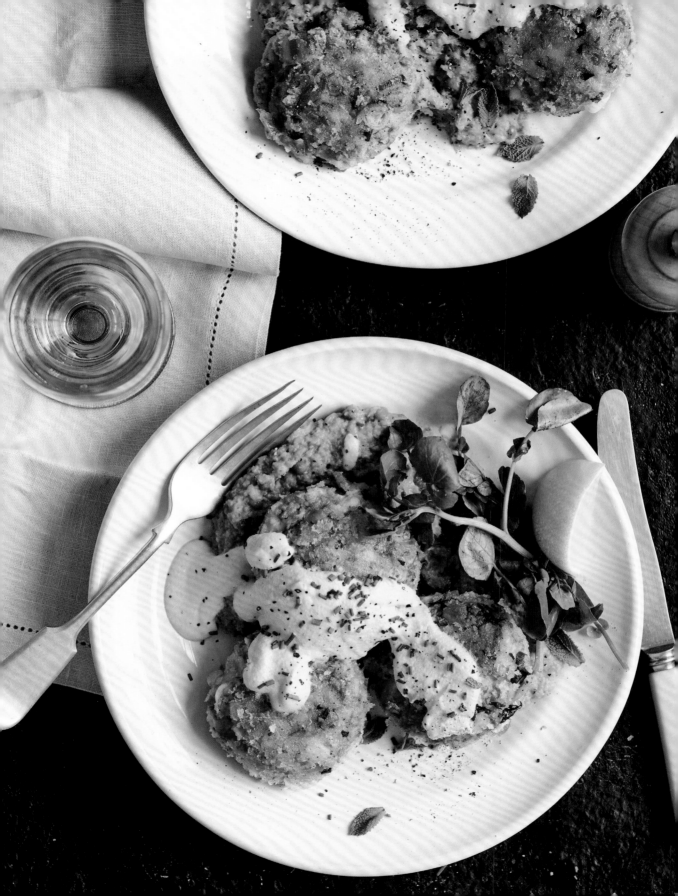

PRAWN LINGUINE AND GARLIC CIABATTA

This one's a goody. It's got bite, zip, heat, sweetness and it's really satisfying. Not only is it delicious, but if you plate it up with a little care and artistry, there's an opportunity to make it look really good too. Definitely one to impress your mates with!

SERVES 4

FOR THE CIABATTA
1 garlic bulb
15g fresh flat-leaf parsley
50g plant-based butter
1 large ciabatta loaf
nooch (nutritional yeast)
    (optional)
sea salt and black pepper

FOR THE PASTA
240g baby plum tomatoes
1 onion
4 garlic cloves
2 fresh red chillies
30g fresh flat-leaf parsley
400g dried linguine (or 500g
    if not using ciabatta)
drizzle of olive oil
20 plant-based prawns
200ml plant-based
    white wine
100g passata
50g rocket
½ lemon
nori sprinkles (optional)
sea salt and black pepper

Preheat oven to 180°C • Food processor • Baking sheet lined with baking parchment • Large saucepan • Fine grater or microplane • Kettle boiled • Tongs • Large frying pan

Prepare the garlic bread • Slice the top off the garlic bulb, then wrap the bulb in foil, adding a good pinch of salt, and bake in the oven for 20–25 minutes • Remove from the oven and allow to cool, then squeeze out the roasted garlic into a food processor, add the parsley and butter and pulse into garlic butter • Taste and season with salt and pepper • Halve the ciabatta and spread with the herby garlic butter • Put the ciabatta in the oven on a baking sheet for 10–15 minutes until nicely toasted

Prepare the pasta water • Bring a large saucepan of salted water to the boil

Prepare the vegetables and herbs • Halve the tomatoes • Peel and dice the onion • Peel and grate the garlic • Finely dice the chillies • Chop the parsley

Cook the pasta • Twist the pasta into the water (using two hands, twist the pasta so it creates a hourglass-like shape into the pan) and cook according to the packet instructions

Prepare the sauce • Heat the olive oil in a large frying pan over a medium heat, add the onion, chillies and garlic and fry for a few minutes until softened • Add the prawns and tomatoes and fry for 2 minutes • Deglaze the pan with the white wine, add the passata and cook until the liquid content has reduced by about a third as you still want it nice and saucy to coat the pasta • If it reduces too quickly, add a few spoonfuls of pasta water to thin it down again

Build the dish • Once cooked, lift the pasta from the cooking water with tongs and transfer to the large frying pan • Sprinkle over half the rocket and chopped parsley, season with salt, pepper and juice from the half lemon (catching any pips in your free hand) and toss to combine • Divide the pasta among 4 large pasta bowls, dress with parsley, the remaining rocket and a sprinkle of nori (if using) • Plate up the garlic bread, sprinkle over some nooch (if using) and serve immediately with the pasta

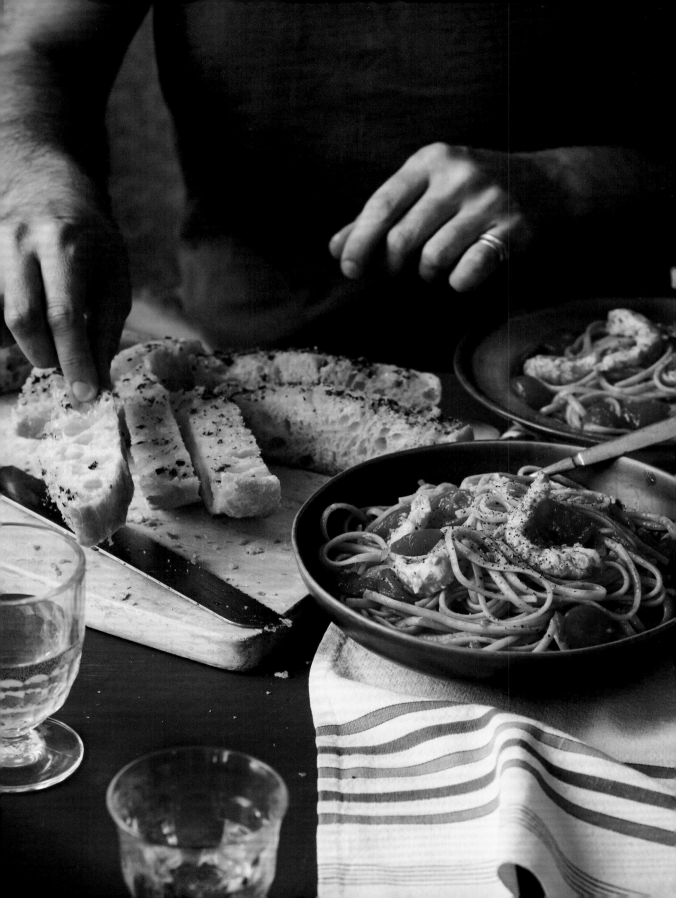

SHRIMP PO'BOY (FRIED SHRIMP SANDWICH)

There are sandwiches and then there are sandwiches. This is a sandwich. In fact, this might be THE sandwich. Crispy and creamy and fresh and satisfying. This is everything you want a sandwich to be. Serve with golden fries, cold cola and bright sunshine to maximise your first Po'Boy experience!

SERVES 4

FOR THE CAJUN SPICE MIX
2½ tsp paprika
2 tsp sea salt
2 tsp garlic powder
1¼ tsp dried oregano
1¼ tsp dried thyme
1 tsp ground black pepper
1 tsp onion powder
1 tsp cayenne pepper
½ tsp dried chilli flakes

FOR THE REMOULADE
1 garlic clove
300g plant-based
   mayonnaise
60g Dijon mustard
1 tbsp paprika
2 tsp Cajun spice mix
   (above)
2 tsp wasabi paste
1 tsp pickle juice from a jar
   of pickled gherkins
1 tsp Louisiana-style hot
   sauce

FOR THE PRAWNS
600g plant-based prawns
180g plain flour
120g fine polenta
3 tbsp Cajun spice mix
   (above)
250g plain dairy-free
   yoghurt
1 litre vegetable
   or sunflower oil
sea salt and black pepper

TO SERVE
4 small French sticks
1 beef tomato
1 large baby gem (or 2 small)
4 gherkins
hot sauce

Fine grater or microplane • Whisk • Baking sheet lined with baking parchment • Large saucepan • Slotted spoon or spider

Make the Cajun spice mix • Stir all the spices together in a bowl and set aside (try to use fresh jars of spices – avoiding anything that's been at the back of your cupboards for a while – as this will keep the flavours popping)

Make the remoulade • Peel the garlic and grate it into a mixing bowl • Add all the remaining ingredients and whisk to combine • Set aside in the fridge in a suitable container

Prepare the prawns • Put the prawns in a bowl and season with salt and pepper • In a separate bowl, mix the flour and polenta together and set aside • Add 3 tablespoons of the Cajun spice mix to a bowl with the yoghurt and whisk • Dip some of the prawns in the yoghurt mix, shake off any excess, then dip into the flour mix, making sure the prawns are well coated • Transfer the coated prawns to a lined baking sheet and repeat until all the prawns are coated • Pour the frying oil in a large saucepan and heat over a medium heat

Prepare the remaining ingredients • Slice the bread in half and remove a little of the soft bread inside to make space for the prawns • Slice the beef tomato • Trim, core and shred the lettuce • Slice the gherkins • Spread the bread with remoulade and fill with lettuce, tomato slices and gherkin

Cook the prawns • Check the oil temperature (it needs to be 180°C) in the pan and start to fry the prawns in batches for 2–3 minutes per batch, until crisp and nicely browned, removing them with a slotted spoon or spider and draining onto kitchen paper each time • Check the temperature of the oil is 180°C before frying each batch • When the shrimp is ready, load the po'boys up and serve with a little extra remoulade and a drizzle of hot sauce

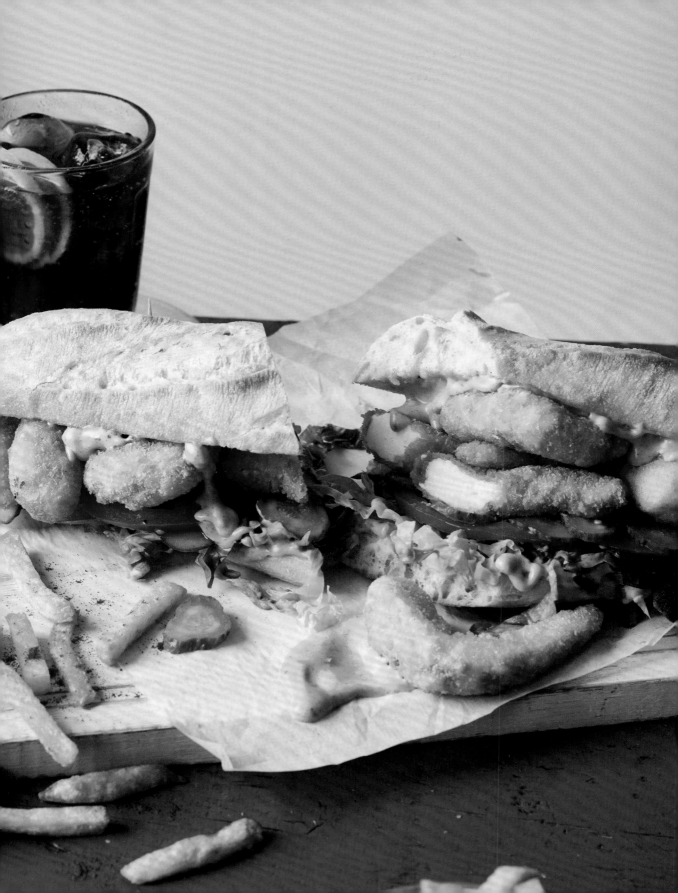

SEAFOOD PAELLA

Paella is a dish that's really easy to get wrong, which is why we spent a long while getting this one just right. One of the best things about a good paella is that every forkful is different from the last. Pops of freshness, hints of zippiness, bursts of aroma... It's a rainbow of flavours and we have our fingers firmly crossed that you and your family appreciate it as much as we do.

SERVES 4

500g paella rice

FOR THE CALDO (PAELLA BROTH)
2 carrots
1 onion
1 medium bunch Swiss chard
100g green beans
2 rosemary sprigs
splash of olive oil
1 tbsp sweet smoked paprika
2.5 litres vegetable stock

FOR THE CONFIT TOMATO
4 large tomatoes
200ml olive oil
pinch of saffron strands
½ tsp sweet paprika
sea salt

FOR THE TOPPING
4 king oyster mushrooms
1 x 400g tin banana blossom
250g asparagus spears
8 plant-based prawns

Stock pot • Frying pan • Sieve • Large skillet or paella pan (ideally 40cm diameter) • Wooden spoon • Measuring jug • Ladle

Make the caldo • Peel and thinly slice the carrots and onion • Roughly chop the Swiss chard and beans • Remove the needles from the rosemary sprigs and finely chop • Warm the olive oil in a stock pot over a medium heat, add the onion and carrots and fry for 3–4 minutes • Add the paprika and vegetable stock to the pot • Add the chard, rosemary and green beans to the pan and simmer over a low heat for 30 minutes • Take the pot off the heat and leave to steep (allow the flavours to develop) until you're ready to cook

Make the confit tomato • Roughly chop the tomatoes • Warm the olive oil in a frying pan over a medium heat • Add the tomatoes, saffron, paprika and a large pinch of salt to the pan, stir to combine and leave to simmer for about 30 minutes until the liquid has reduced • Pour the tomatoes through a sieve into a bowl to separate the oil and the tomatoes • Transfer the tomatoes to another bowl and set both to one side

Make the paella • Warm 80ml of the reserved tomato oil in a large skillet or paella pan over a medium heat, add the paella rice and 100g of the confit tomato and stir to coat • Add half the caldo to the pan with a ladle, passing it through a sieve to catch any sediment • Once the rice is just submerged in the caldo, cook over a medium-high heat for 10 minutes

Prepare the toppings • Cut the king oyster mushrooms into 1cm-thick scallop-shaped discs and cross-hatch the face of each disc with a sharp knife • Drain the banana blossom, rinse off the brine and cut into bite-sized pieces • Trim the asparagus • Fry the toppings (including the prawns) in a frying pan with the remaining tomato oil over a medium heat for 2–3 minutes until cooked through (refer to the cooking time on the prawn packet for guidance)

Finish the paella and serve • Season the mushroom scallops, banana blossom, prawns and asparagus, and stir some of them into the paella, place the rest on top of the paella • Add ladles of the remaining caldo to the paella gradually every time the rice looks like it's absorbed the liquid until all the caldo is used up and the rice has swollen and cooked through – this will take about 10 minutes • Spoon the paella onto plates and serve immediately

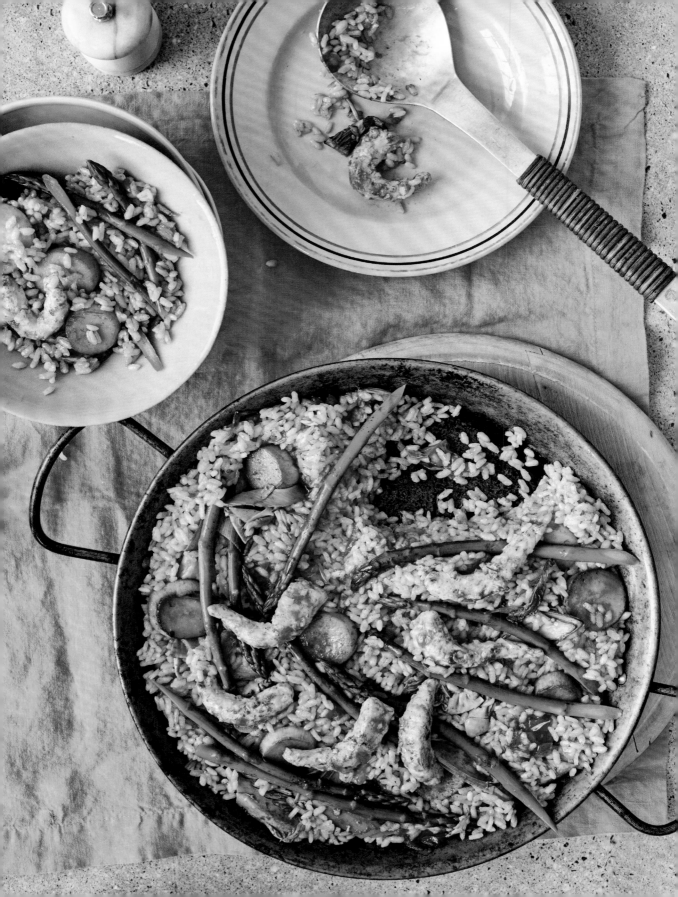

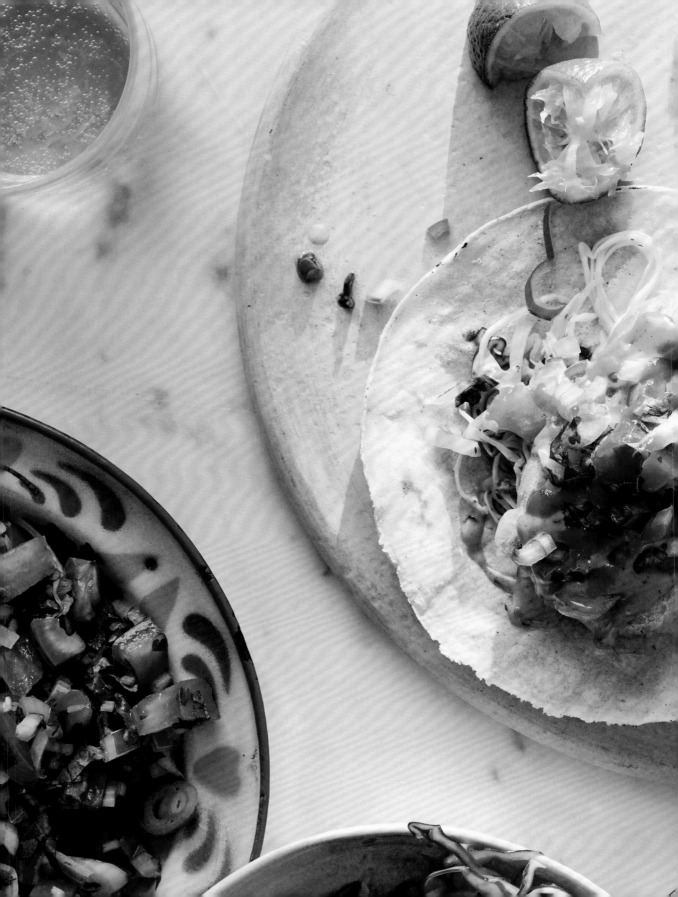

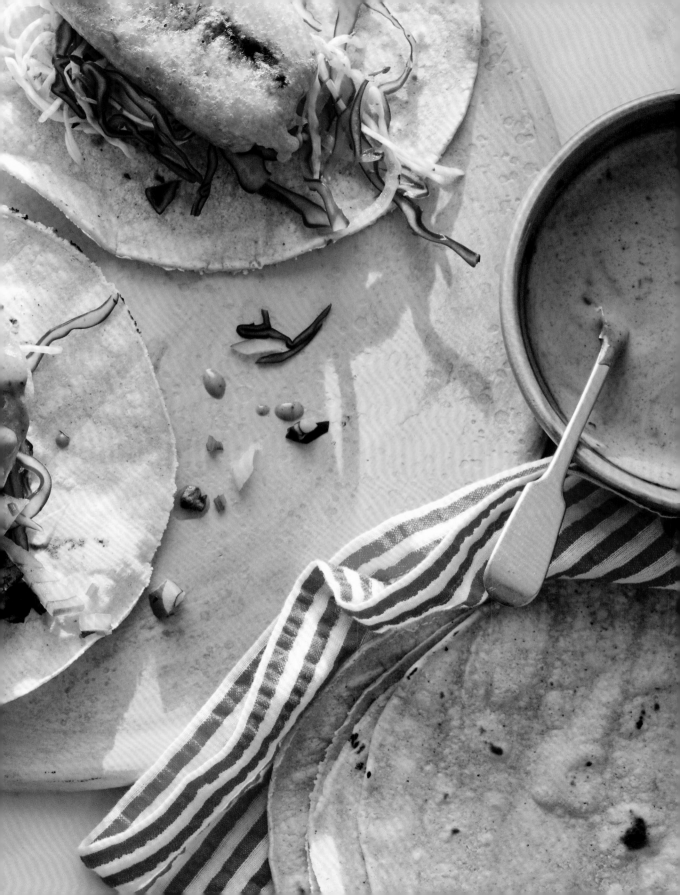

CHEESE

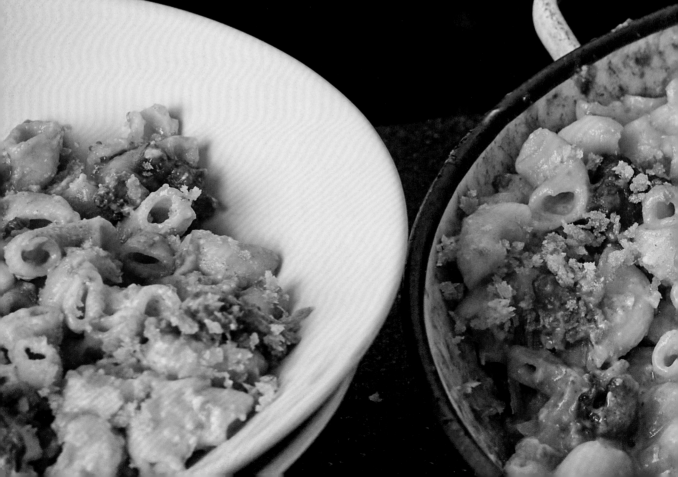

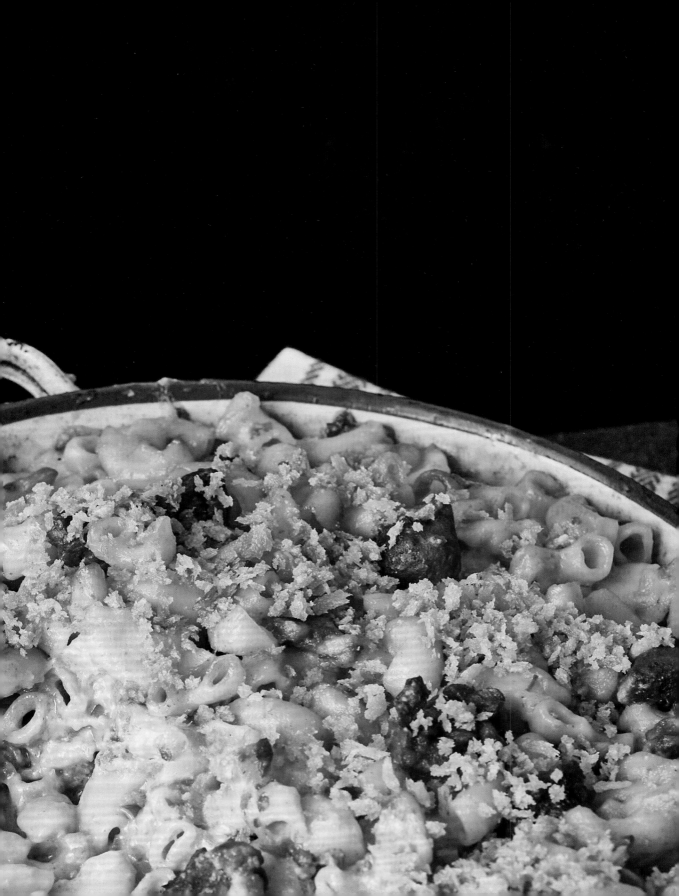

BACON CAULIFLOWER CHEESE

Super cheesy, kinda smoky and with just the right amount of saltiness. This is a cracking cauliflower recipe that's great as part of a roast dinner or served as a main with some steamed veggies. The sauce has a rich cheesy flavour and melts over the cauliflower and bacon to create a super-stringy coating, topped with crispy breadcrumbs for the perfect veggie-packed recipe. A truly lovely dish that you'll come back to time and time again.

**SERVES 4 AS A MAIN,
6 AS A SIDE**

FOR THE BASE
1 onion
2 garlic cloves
drizzle of olive oil
2 x 120g packs plant-
    based bacon
sea salt

FOR THE CAULIFLOWER
2 heads of cauliflower (or
    1 very large cauliflower)
drizzle of olive oil
sea salt and black pepper

FOR THE SAUCE
100g plant-based butter
100g tapioca flour
100g nooch (nutritional
    yeast)
100ml plant-based cream
1 tbsp Dijon mustard
600ml unsweetened
    almond milk
1 lemon
sea salt

FOR THE TOPPING
2 slices of bread
    (sourdough ideally)
2 tbsp nooch (nutritional
    yeast)
2 tbsp olive oil
2 spring onions
sea salt and black pepper

Preheat oven to 190°C • Large frying pan • Large baking tray • Whisk
• Blender

Make the base • Peel and thinly slice the onion and peel and finely dice the garlic cloves • Heat a little drizzle of olive oil in a large frying pan over a medium heat • Add the sliced onion, diced garlic and a small pinch of salt • Mix well and cook for 5–10 minutes, or until the onion softens • Cut the bacon into small cubes and add to the pan • Mix well and cook for another 5 minutes

Cook the cauliflower • Cut the cauliflower into small florets and place on a large baking tray • Add the cooked onion and garlic mixture to the tray and mix well until everything is well combined • Add another drizzle of olive oil, a small pinch each of salt and pepper and mix well until everything is coated in the oil (be careful not to over-season the cauliflower as the bacon will provide most of the saltiness you need) • Cook in the oven for 15 minutes

Make the sauce • Place the pan you used to cook the onion and bacon base back over a medium heat and add the butter • Once melted, add the tapioca flour and cook for 5 minutes, stirring constantly • Remove from the heat, add the nooch, cream, Dijon mustard and start gradually adding the almond milk, stirring constantly • Add a good pinch of salt • Halve the lemon and squeeze in the juice from both halves, catching any pips in your free hand • Whisk the sauce over the heat for 5–10 minutes until there are no lumps in the mixture and it comes together to form a smooth, creamy sauce

Make the topping • Blitz the bread to breadcrumbs in a blender, then stir in the nooch and olive oil with a pinch of salt

Finish the dish • Turn the oven up to 210°C • After 15 minutes, remove the cauliflower from the oven and pour in the sauce • Mix well until all of the sauce is mixed through the cauliflower • Top with the breadcrumbs and place back in the oven for another 10–15 minutes until the top turns golden brown

Time to serve • Trim and slice the spring onions for the topping • Once the top has turned golden brown, remove from the oven and sprinkle with some slices of spring onions and freshly ground black pepper

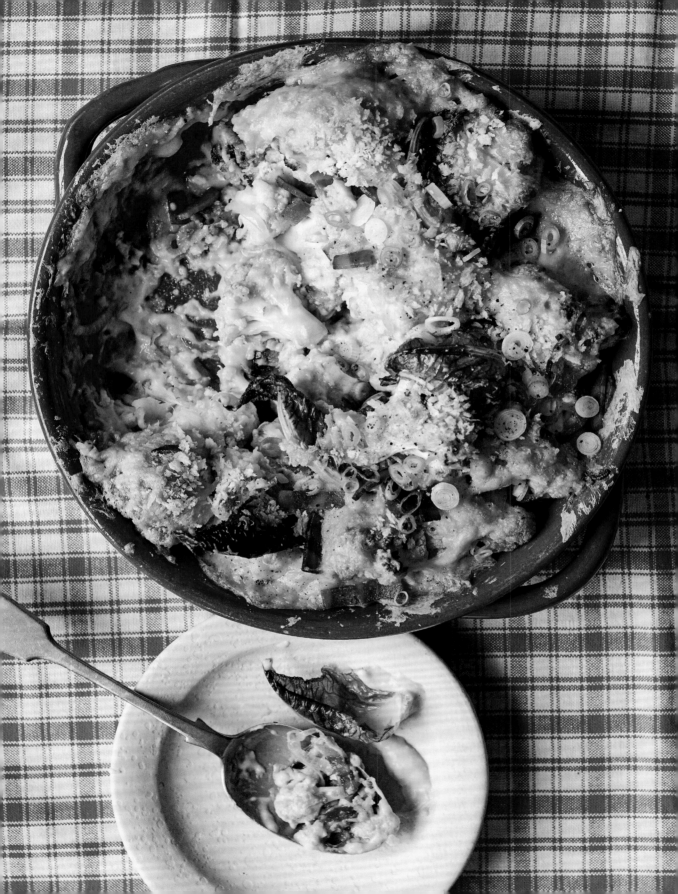

CHEESE AND MUSHROOM OMELETTE

We think that if 'luncheon' is the formal word for 'lunch', then 'bruncheon' should be the formal word for 'brunch'. Now that we've got that out of the way, we think you should make this recipe for bruncheon as soon as you can!

SERVES 2

FOR THE MUSHROOMS
100g button mushrooms
1 tbsp light soy sauce
5 drops of liquid smoke (optional)
1 tbsp olive oil

FOR THE OMELETTES
1 x 300g pack silken tofu
2 tbsp cornflour
4 tbsp plain flour
4 tbsp nooch (nutritional yeast)
pinch of turmeric, optional
8 cherry tomatoes
2 tbsp plant-based butter (for cooking)
100g grated plant-based cheddar
sea salt and black pepper

TO SERVE
handful of chives
2 spring onions

Preheat oven to 200°C • Baking tray • Powerful blender • Medium frying pan

Cook the mushrooms • Thinly slice the mushrooms and spoon into a mixing bowl • Add the soy sauce, liquid smoke (if using) and olive oil • Mix well to ensure all of the mushrooms are coated in the liquid • Spread out on a baking tray and bake in the oven for 7–8 minutes until golden and crisp • Once cooked, remove from the oven and set aside until needed

Make the omelette mixture • Drain the tofu and place it in a powerful blender along with the cornflour, plain flour, nooch and turmeric (if using) • Blend until a smooth batter forms • Season with salt and pepper • Cut the tomatoes into small pieces

Prepare the ingredients to serve • Thinly slice the chives and trim and slice the spring onions

Cook the omelettes • Heat 1 tablespoon of the butter in a frying pan over a medium heat • Once melted, add half of the tofu mixture and spread it out in the pan • Cook for 1–2 minutes, until slightly setting, then scatter over half of the mushrooms, chopped tomatoes, and grated cheese • Cook for 3 more minutes, until the mixture has set, then flip one side over the other to create a half-moon shape • Slide onto a plate and repeat this process to make the second omelette

Time to serve • Scatter the omelettes with the chives and spring onions before serving

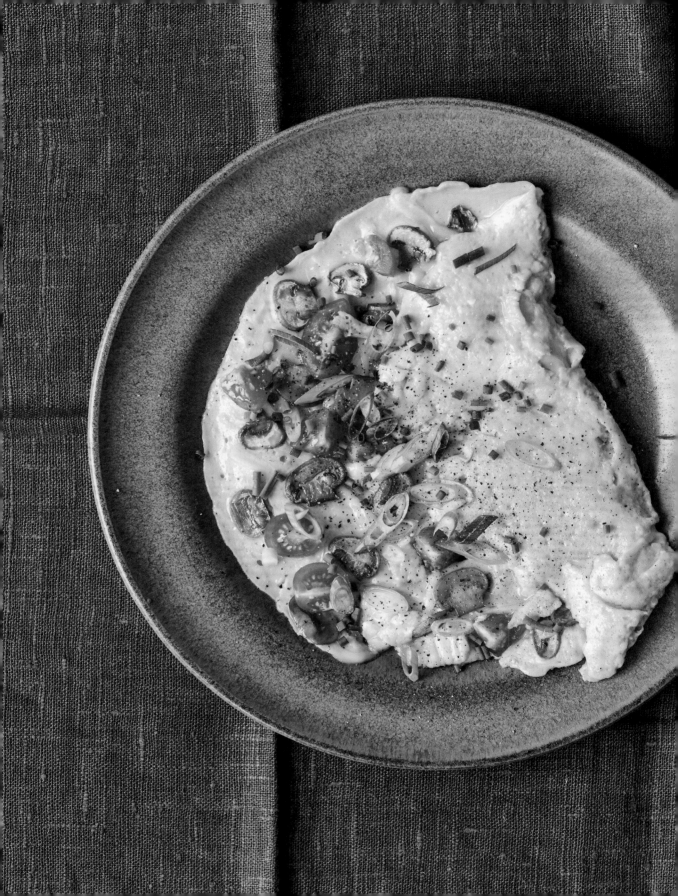

CHORIZO MAC AND CHEESE

Chorizo? Good. Cheese? Good. Pasta? Good. When you blend these three elements together, you're left with good to the power of three. Triple good. Echalion shallots are cooked down with spiced plant-based chorizo sausages and paprika before being mixed with plant-based cheese and oat milk to create a deliciously cheesy sauce that coats the macaroni pasta. We top the whole dish with seasoned breadcrumbs for an extra crispy crunch.

SERVES 4–6 AS A MAIN, 8 AS A SIDE

FOR THE MAC AND CHEESE
2 echalion shallots
2 tsp sea salt
1 tbsp olive oil
2 tsp garlic purée
220g plant-based
    chorizo sausages
1 tsp smoked paprika
500g macaroni pasta
20g plant-based butter
40g plain flour
500ml unsweetened oat milk
200g plant-based
    grated cheddar
10g nooch (nutritional yeast)

FOR THE BREADCRUMBS
2 tbsp olive oil
50g breadcrumbs (or
    bread, blitzed to crumbs)
pinch of sea salt
1 tsp ground black pepper
½ tsp smoked paprika

Preheat oven to 200°C • Ovenproof high-sided frying pan • Small frying pan • Kettle boiled • Large saucepan • Colander

Cook the chorizo • Peel and thinly slice the shallots • Place the slices in a colander and season with the salt • Warm the olive oil in a high-sided frying pan over a medium heat • Add the shallots and stir for 1 minute • Add the garlic purée and stir for a further minute • Crumble the chorizo sausages into the pan (removing the skin) and fry for 5–6 minutes until the sausages are starting to crisp up and the shallot is golden • Sprinkle over the smoked paprika, stir for 1 minute, transfer to a plate and set to one side (don't clean out the pan)

Fry the breadcrumbs • Warm the olive oil in small frying pan over a medium heat • Add the breadcrumbs, salt, pepper and smoked paprika and fry for 4–5 minutes until golden and crispy • Set to one side

Cook the pasta • Cook the pasta in a large saucepan of salted boiling water over a high heat according to the packet instructions

Make the cheese sauce • Add the butter to the high-sided frying pan and melt over a medium heat • Sprinkle the flour into the pan and stir to make a roux • Pour the oat milk into the pan, stirring constantly, until gently simmering and cook for a few minutes until thickened • Add the plant-based cheese and nooch to the pan and stir until melted

Finish the dish and serve • Add the cooked pasta to the sauce and stir to combine • Add the chorizo to the pan and fold into the saucy pasta • Sprinkle over the breadcrumbs, put the pan in the oven and roast for 10–15 minutes (if you don't have an ovenproof high-sided frying pan, transfer the mixture to a baking dish before sprinkling over the breadcrumbs) • Take the pan out of the oven, spoon the mac and cheese into bowls and serve immediately with a little side salad

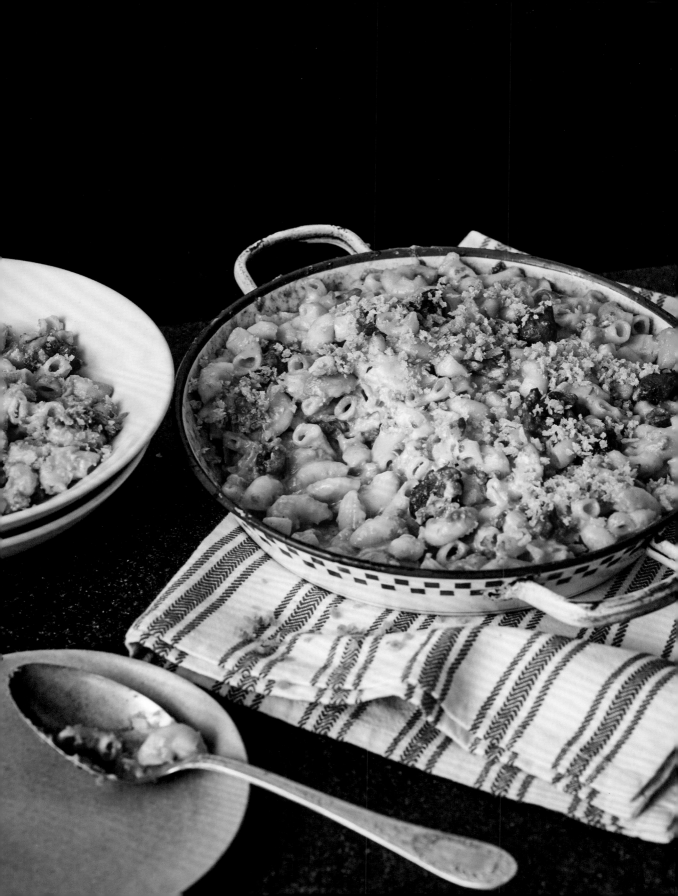

SPANAKOPITA WITH TOMATO AND POMEGRANATE ZA'ATAR SALAD

This recipe uses a truck-full of spinach but it's worth it – the spinach wilts down and is blended together with cashews, plant-based feta, silken tofu, fresh mint, dill and parsley to create the silky smooth green base layer. It's then topped with crunchy filo pastry to make the most delicious dish that everyone will love.

SERVES 4

FOR THE SPANAKOPITA
1 red onion
3 garlic cloves
½ leek
4 spring onions
100g raw unsalted cashews
200ml boiling water
390g spinach
2 tbsp olive oil, plus extra
    for brushing
200g plant-based
    feta cheese
½ tsp ground or grated
    nutmeg
80g plant-based
    parmesan
1 lemon
15g fresh dill
10g fresh mint
5g fresh oregano
10g fresh flat-leaf parsley
300g silken tofu
40g pine nuts
250g plant-based filo pastry
salt

FOR THE TOMATO SALAD
50g freekeh
2 echalion shallots
12 tomatoes of different
    sizes and colours
handful of pomegranate
    seeds
4 tbsp olive oil
2 tbsp pomegranate
    molasses
2 tbsp red wine vinegar
1 tsp za'atar
1 tsp sea salt

Preheat oven to 200°C • Frying pan • Tongs • Powerful blender • Fine grater or microplane • 30 x 25cm baking tin • Saucepan • Pastry brush

Prepare the ingredients • Peel and dice the onion and garlic • Trim and thinly slice the leek and spring onions • Place the cashews in a heatproof bowl, cover with the boiling water and set aside for at least 30 minutes to soften • Wash the spinach then wilt it in a dry frying pan over a medium heat, turning it with tongs • Once wilted, set aside until needed

Make the filling • Place the pan you used for wilting the spinach over a medium heat and add the olive oil • Add the onion, garlic, leeks and a pinch of salt • Mix well and cook for 5–10 minutes until soft • Remove from the heat and stir through the spring onions • Spoon into a large bowl and set aside • Drain the cashews and spoon into a powerful blender with a little of the soaking water, along with the feta, nutmeg, parmesan cheese, the juice and grated zest of the lemon and all of the fresh herbs • Drain the silken tofu and add it the blender with a pinch of salt • Blend until the mixture comes together but is still a little chunky, adding more of the soaking water if needed • Spoon the mixture into the mixing bowl with the cooked onions • Squeeze the water from the spinach and finely chop • Mix the chopped spinach though the mixture, along with the pine nuts

Assemble the dish • Brush the baking tin with olive oil • Line the tin with half the filo pastry, brushing each sheet with oil as you go and taking care not to press them down in the process • Leave any excess filo pastry overhanging the sides • Spoon the filling into the baking tin and level the top using the back of a spoon • Scrunch the remaining pastry sheets and place them on top of the pie filling • Fold the overhanging bottom layers of filo pastry inwards

Cook the dish • Bake in the oven for 20 minutes, then turn the heat down to 160°C and cook for a final 10 minutes, or until golden

Make the tomato salad • Place a saucepan over a medium heat and add the freekeh • Cover with just enough water to cover the freekeh and simmer over a medium heat for 15–20 minutes • Peel and thinly slice the shallots • Slice the tomatoes into thin circles and scatter them over a serving plate • Sprinkle over the shallots, pomegranate seeds and freekeh • Drizzle over the olive oil, pomegranate molasses, red wine vinegar, za'atar and salt

Time to serve • Remove the dish from the oven and leave to cool slightly before serving in the middle of the table, alongside the tomato salad

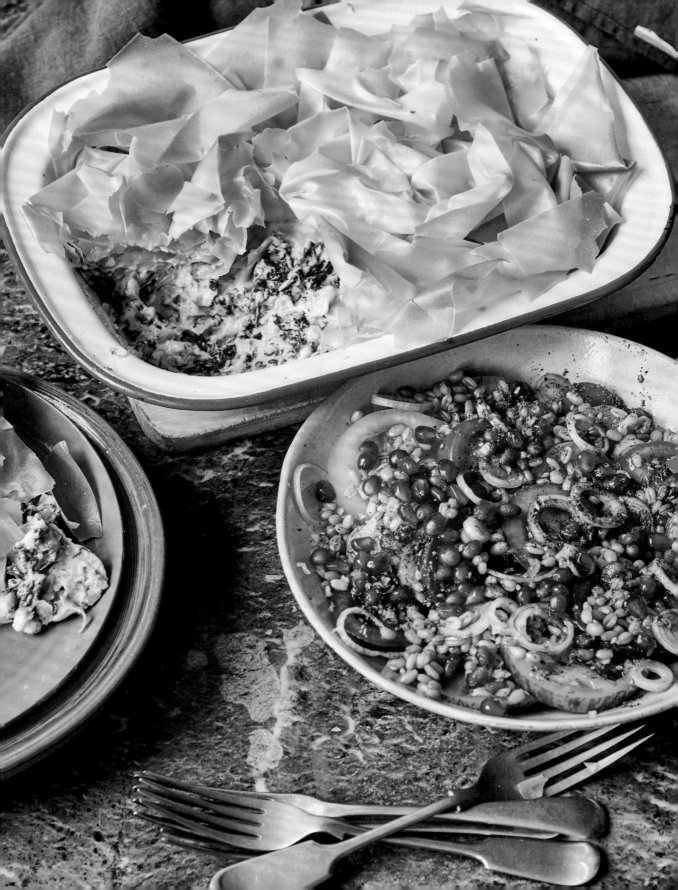

QUATTRO FORMAGGI LASAGNE

We love lasagne, you love lasagne, our mates love lasagne, your mates love lasagne, our families love lasagne, your family loves lasagne. We reckon everyone loves lasagne and, what's more, we reckon everyone is gonna love THIS lasagne because it's head-scratchingly delicious. Make one, get your mates over and get stuck in! It freezes well, too.

SERVES 8

350g dried plant-based
    lasagne sheets

FOR THE RAGU
2 brown onions
2 carrots
2 celery sticks
2 garlic cloves
1kg chestnut mushrooms
50ml olive oil
1 tsp dried chilli flakes
150ml plant-based red wine
2 x 400g tins chopped
    tomatoes
50g plant-based bacon
450g plant-based mince
sea salt and black pepper

FOR THE BÉCHAMEL
60g plain flour
50g nooch (nutritional
    yeast)
800ml unsweetened
    almond milk
100g plant-based cheddar
100g plant-based feta
    cheese
100g plant-based smoked
    cheddar
30g plant-based parmesan

FOR THE SIMPLE SALAD
1 lemon
100ml extra-virgin olive oil
1 head radicchio
1 head baby gem lettuce
1 head butter lettuce
15g fresh basil leaves
15g fresh mint leaves
sea salt and black pepper

Food processor • Large saucepan • Large frying pan • Preheat oven to 180°C • Medium saucepan • Whisk • Box grater • Lasagne dish (25 x 35cm)

Prepare the base ingredients • Peel and roughly chop the onions and carrots and trim the celery • Peel the garlic • Halve the mushrooms and put them in the food processor with the onions, carrots, celery and garlic and pulse to create a mince

Start the ragu • Warm 30ml of the olive oil in a large saucepan over a medium heat, add the onion, carrot, celery, garlic and chilli flakes to the pan with a pinch of salt and fry for 5–6 minutes until soft, stirring occasionally • Add the mushrooms to the pan, stir to combine and sweat for further 5–6 minutes to cook off most of the liquid content of the mushrooms • Add the red wine and simmer for 3–4 minutes to cook off the alcohol • Add the chopped tomatoes, stir and simmer gently for 10 minutes, or until the liquid has reduced

Finish the ragu • Dice the bacon • Warm the remaining olive oil in a large frying pan over a medium-high heat, break in the mince and fry for 3–4 minutes to caramelise and brown • Spoon the mince into the sauce, add the bacon to the frying pan and fry for 2–3 minutes before stirring that into the sauce too • Taste and season to perfection with salt and pepper

Prepare the béchamel • Put the flour and nooch in a medium saucepan, put the pan over a medium heat and gradually whisk in the milk until smooth then cook for 5–10 minutes until it's thick and creamy • Put the lid on the pan and set to one side (you may need to add a splash more milk and whisk once more when it's time to build the lasagne)

Prepare the cheese • Grate the cheeses into a bowl and set to one side

Assemble the lasagne • Spoon a quarter of ragu into the lasagne dish and spread over the bottom • Top with a single layer of lasagne sheets, breaking the sheets where necessary to achieve a tight fit • Spoon a quarter of béchamel over the pasta and smooth out • Evenly sprinkle a quarter of all the cheeses over the béchamel • Repeat this process, ensuring you finish with a layer of béchamel and cheese • Place the lasagne in the oven and bake for 50 minutes

Prepare the simple salad • Halve the lemon and squeeze it into a large bowl, catching any pips in your free hand • Add the extra-virgin olive oil, season to taste and whisk to combine • Pick, trim, wash and drain the radicchio and lettuce leaves • Add the lettuce and herbs to the bowl and toss to combine and coat

Time to serve • Check the lasagne – if you think it could do with a little more colour on top, grill it for a couple of minutes • Take the lasagne out of the oven and leave to rest for a couple of minutes before cutting into slices, transferring to plates and serving with the simple salad

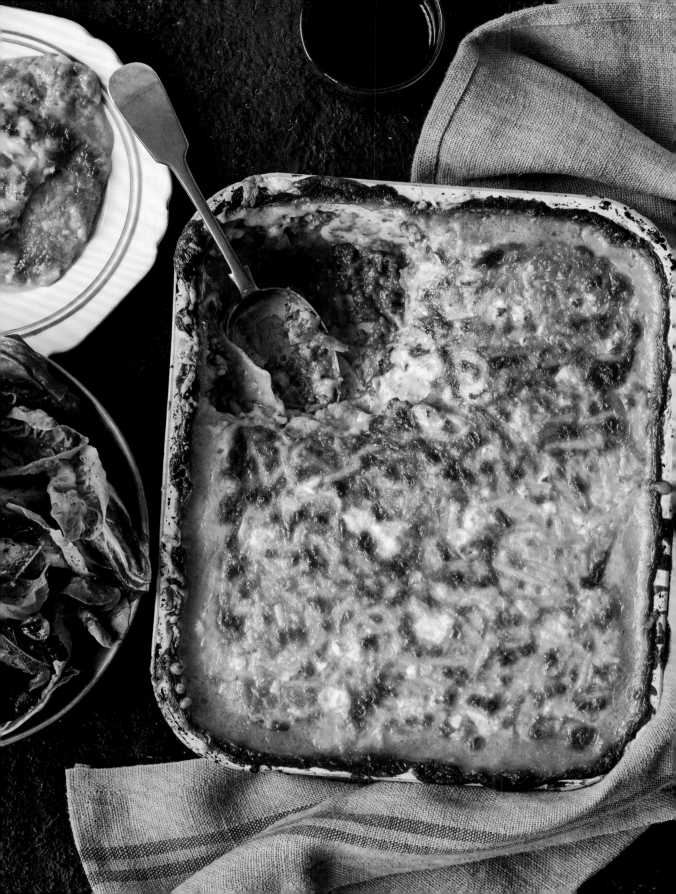

HEARTY HALLOUMI SALAD

If you ask us, salads should have big, punchy flavours and a robust, satisfying bite; they should please your palate and your stomach in equal measure. This salad does both of those things perfectly. Rustle it up in warmer months, serve with a cold glass of good white wine, and you will not be disappointed.

SERVES 4

FOR THE HALLOUMI
1 x 325g block firm tofu
3 lemons
3 tbsp olive oil
3 tbsp nooch (nutritional yeast)
2 tsp dried mint
½ tsp garlic powder
sea salt

FOR THE SALAD
2 red onions
drizzle of olive oil
2 vegetable stock pots
600ml boiling water
2 red peppers
250g cherry tomatoes
200g pearl barley
handful of fresh mint leaves
1 bag of mixed leaves (about 150g)
1 lemon
sea salt

Baking sheet lined with baking parchment • Large saucepan • Heatproof jug • Griddle pan

Prepare the halloumi • Press the tofu to drain off any liquid • Cut the lemons in half and squeeze the juice into a container, catching any pips in your free hand • Add the olive oil, nooch, dried mint, garlic powder and a pinch of salt and stir to form a smooth paste • Cut the tofu into 8 strips • Put the tofu strips in the container and coat in the marinade • Leave to marinate in the fridge for at least 2 hours • Preheat oven to 180°C after 2 hours' marinating time

Bake the halloumi • Remove the halloumi from the marinade and bake it in the oven on the lined baking sheet for 25 minutes

While the halloumi is baking, make the salad • Peel the red onions and slice them thickly • Place a large saucepan over a medium heat and add a drizzle of olive oil • Once warm, add the onion slices and a pinch of salt, mix well and cook for about 10 minutes until the onion softens • Mix the vegetable stock pots with the boiling water in a heatproof jug • Trim, halve and core the red peppers, cut into small cubes and halve the tomatoes • Add the peppers to the onions and cook for another 5 minutes before adding the pearl barley and hot vegetable stock • Cook the pearl barley according to the packet instructions until the barley has absorbed all the water and becomes soft

Griddle the halloumi • Warm a griddle pan over a medium-high heat, lay the marinated tofu strips on the pan and sear for 2 minutes on each side to create lovely dark griddle lines • Transfer the halloumi to a plate and season with a good pinch of salt

Build the salad and serve • Remove the pearl barley from the heat, slice the mint leaves and mix through the pearl barley, along with the mixed leaves and tomatoes • Halve the lemon and squeeze in the juice from both halves, catching any pips in your free hand • Spoon the salad onto the bottom of a large serving plate and top with the halloumi slices

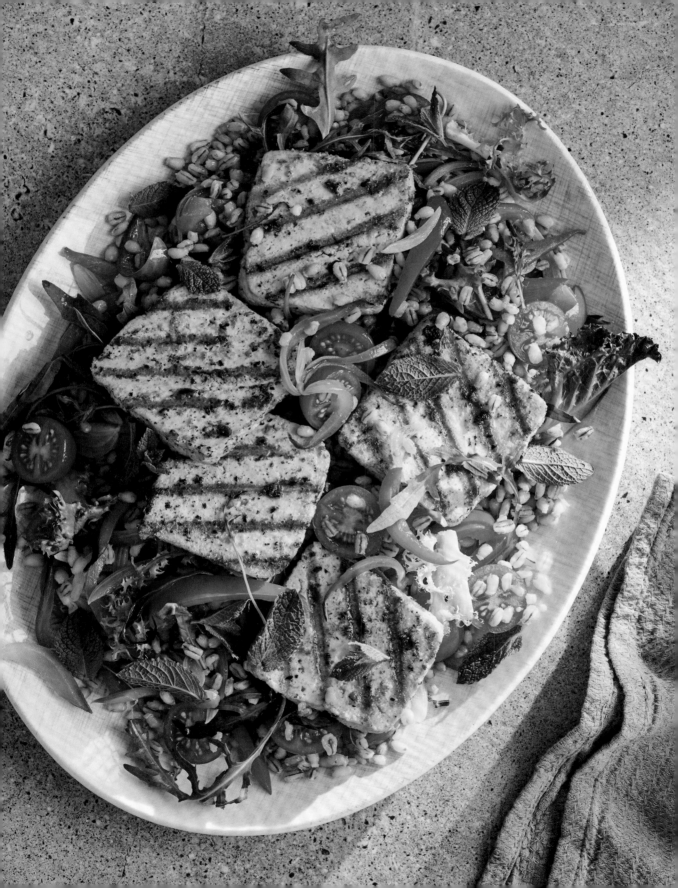

POUTINE

Wikipedia says, 'Poutine is a dish of French fries and cheese curds topped with a brown gravy. It emerged in Quebec, in the late 1950s in the Centre-du-Québec region, though its exact origins are uncertain and there are several competing claims regarding its invention.' We say: 'Chips, cheese and gravy? GO ON THEN!'.

SERVES 4

FOR THE CHIPS
1kg Maris Piper potatoes
vegetable oil or olive oil,
    for frying
sea salt

FOR THE CHEESE CURDS
75g raw unsalted cashews
35ml unsweetened
    almond milk
½ tsp white miso paste
1½ tsp apple cider vinegar
1½ tbsp nooch
    (nutritional yeast)
25g plant-based
    grated parmesan
½ small garlic clove
pinch of sea salt

FOR THE GRAVY
1 vegetable stock pot
300ml boiling water
3 red onions
4 garlic cloves
drizzle of olive oil
3 tbsp tomato purée
400ml plant-based red
    wine (mild flavoured)
3 thyme sprigs
2 large bay leaves
    (or 3 small)
1 tbsp tamari
2 tsp light brown sugar
pinch of sea salt

TO SERVE
handful of fresh
    flat-leaf parsley
pinch of black pepper

2 large saucepans • Kitchen paper • Kettle boiled • Powerful blender • Slotted spoon • Baking tray lined with baking parchment

Start the chips • Cut the potatoes into chips, as thin or as chunky as you like (we like to keep the skins on, but you can remove them if you prefer) • Place the chips in a large saucepan of salted water and bring to the boil over a medium heat • Reduce the heat to low and simmer for 3–6 minutes (depending how chunky your chips are) • After 3–6 minutes, drain and leave to dry on a plate lined with kitchen paper

Start the cheese curds • Place the cashews into a heatproof bowl and cover with boiling water • Leave to one side for at least 20 minutes until needed

Make the gravy • Mix the stock pot with the boiling water until completely dissolved • Peel and roughly slice the onions, and peel and dice the garlic • Place a large saucepan over a medium heat and add the olive oil • Add the onions, garlic and salt • Mix well and cook for 5–10 minutes until the onions start to soften • Add the stock, tomato purée, red wine, thyme sprigs, bay leaves, tamari and sugar • Bring to the boil then reduce the heat to low and simmer for 25 minutes, adding a splash of water if the gravy becomes too thick

Finish the cheese curds • Drain the cashews and spoon into a powerful blender • Add the almond milk, miso paste, apple cider vinegar, nooch, parmesan, garlic and salt • Blend until really thick, smooth and creamy, adding a dash more almond milk if needed • Once smooth, place in the fridge until needed

If frying the chips • Place a large saucepan over a medium heat and add about 4cm of vegetable oil • Heat until the oil feels hot enough to fry – a small piece of bread added in should start to bubble immediately • Once hot enough, add the chips – a few at a time– and cook for 6 minutes until golden brown • Once golden, remove the chips using a slotted spoon and transfer to a plate covered in kitchen paper • Repeat this process until you have cooked all of your chips

If baking the chips • Preheat oven to 200°C • After boiling the chips, softly shake them dry and place onto a large baking tray lined with baking parchment • Drizzle with olive oil and bake for about 40 minutes until golden and crispy

Time to serve • Spoon the chips onto serving plates (or 1 large sharing plate) • Spoon over a good amount of the gravy, removing the bay leaves and thyme sprigs • Use a teaspoon to spoon out chunks of the cashew curd and dollop on different places over the chips • Roughly chop the parsley and sprinkle it over the top with a crack of pepper

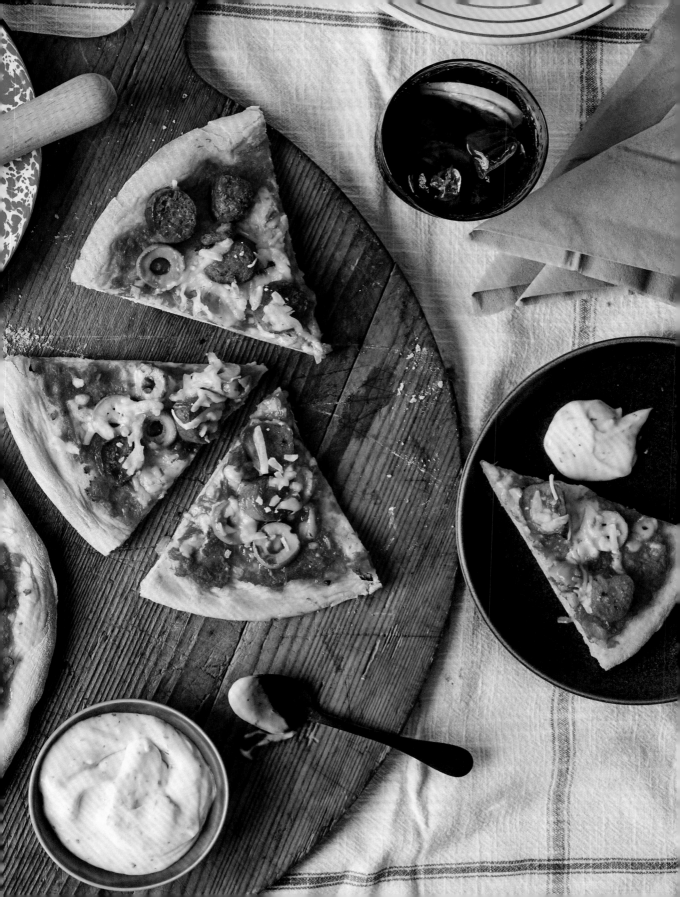

DESSERTS

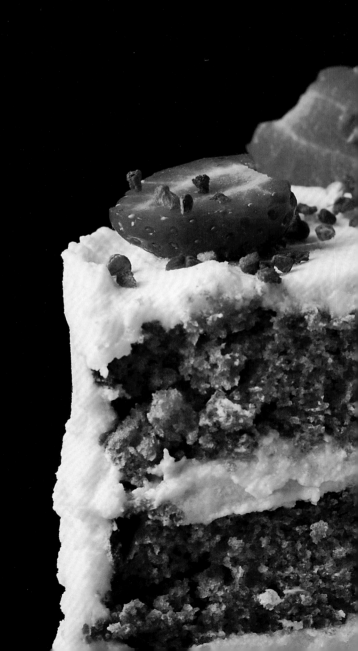

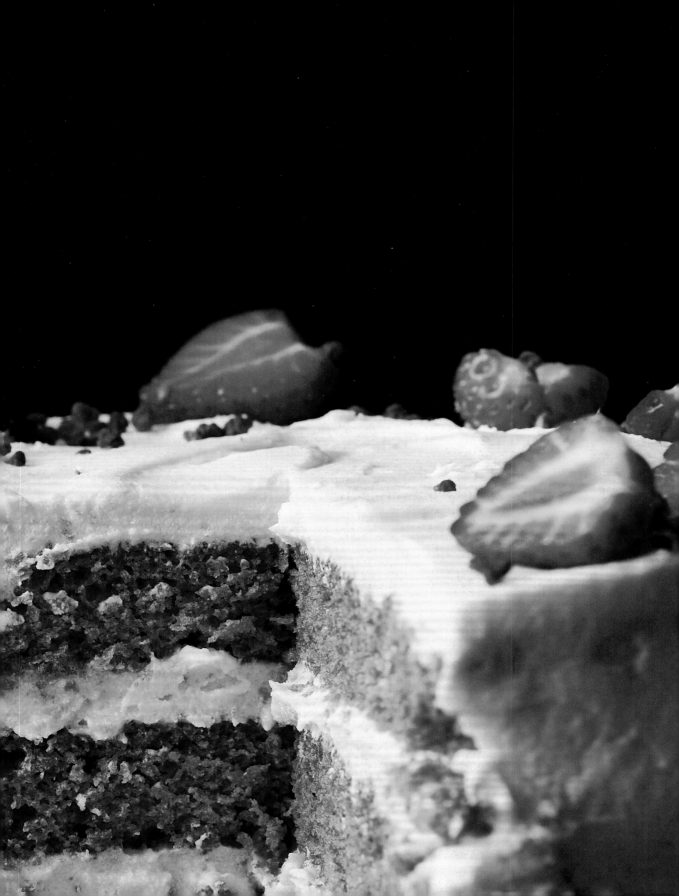

5-MINUTE MUG CAKE

If you fancy a spot of cake to go with your cuppa, you'll be able to rustle up one of these in the time it takes your tea to reach the perfect temperature! A handful of cupboard ingredients, 1 mixing bowl and 80 seconds in the microwave gives you the easiest, gooiest chocolate dessert that makes the perfect sweet treat for 1 (or 2 if you're feeling generous).

SERVES 1

FOR THE CAKE
3 tbsp self-raising flour
3 tbsp caster sugar
1½ tbsp cacao powder
¼ tsp baking powder
⅛ tsp table salt
4 tbsp oat milk
2 tbsp vegetable oil
½ tsp vanilla extract
30g plant-based
   dark chocolate
   (about 3 chunks)

TO SERVE
plant-based ice cream

Large microwavable mug

Make the cake mixture • Put the flour, sugar, cacao powder, baking powder and salt in a large microwaveable mug and mix well using a fork until there are no lumps • Add the oat milk, vegetable oil and vanilla extract and mix again until the mixture comes together and becomes smooth • Place the chocolate pieces on top of the mixture and push into the centre using your finger or the fork so it sinks into the batter

Cook the cake • Place the mug in the microwave and cook for 80 seconds – no longer otherwise it might spill over

Time to serve • Serve the mug cake with a dollop of plant-based ice cream on top

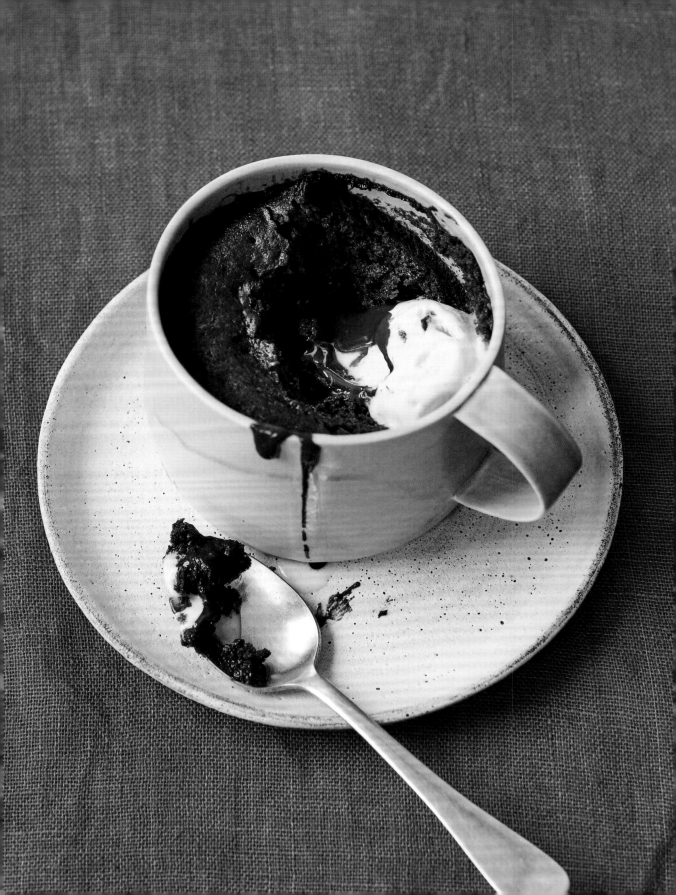

TIRAMISU

Occasionally dishes are brought out of the kitchen at BOSH! HQ that gets the whole team super excited. This is one of those dishes. When this came out, everyone in the office was singing its praises and, to be honest, we're not surprised because it's really, really good. If you like tiramisu and you fancy making one at home, this is the recipe for you. We've made this tiramisu in the traditional way by whipping chickpea water (aquafaba) and sugar together to get a super airy texture before folding through plant-based cream cheese – it makes the most delicious creamy set layers.

SERVES 6-8

5 tbsp espresso powder
250ml boiling water
3 tbsp rum
150g aquafaba (chickpea tin water)
2 tsp cornflour
100g golden caster sugar
500g plant-based cream cheese
2 tbsp icing sugar
1 tsp vanilla extract
400g plant-based biscotti biscuits
1½ tbsp cocoa powder, for dusting

Electric whisk • Deep baking dish about 35 x 30cm • Sieve

Make the coffee liquid • Mix the espresso powder with the boiling water and rum in a heatproof bowl or jug until all the espresso powder has dissolved into the liquid • Leave to cool to room temperature

Make the base • Place the aquafaba into a large bowl and use an electric whisk to whisk the mixture for 5–8 minutes until it turns white, is aerated and forms soft peaks • Combine the cornflour and sugar, then gradually add them to the mixture, continuing to mix for up to 5 minutes until all of the sugar granules have dissolved and the mixture becomes thick • In a separate bowl, whisk (with an electric whisk or hand whisk) the cream cheese, icing sugar and vanilla extract together until they soften a little • Add the cream cheese mixture to the aquafaba mixture and whisk together until smooth and creamy

Dip the biscotti • Dip the biscotti biscuits, one at a time, into the coffee liquid for 2–3 seconds (do not dip them for longer than this)

Assemble the dish • Layer the soaked biscotti biscuits on the bottom of the deep baking dish so they cover the base • Spoon over half of the cream cheese mixture and use a spoon to spread it out so it covers all of the biscotti biscuits • Sift over a thin layer of cocoa powder • Repeat this process with another layer of biscotti biscuits, cream cheese and cocoa powder

Let the dish rest • Place the dish in the fridge and leave to rest for at least 6 hours before serving

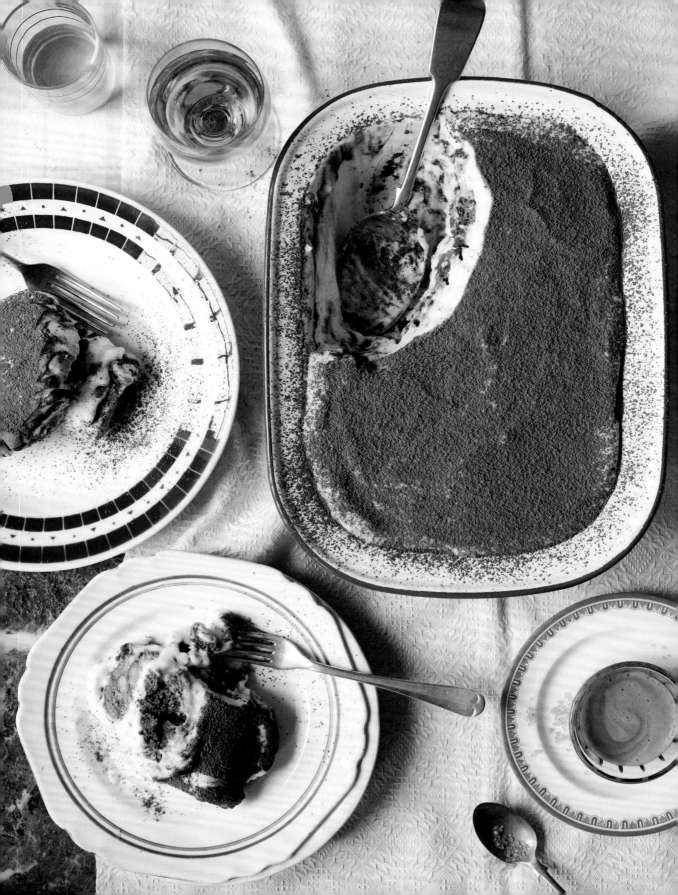

APRICOT TART

This was one of the most popular desserts at BOSH! HQ when we made it during recipe testing – slices of apricots are piled on top of a soft layer of plant-based frangipane, and the whole thing is then glazed with apricot jam for a super-sweet finish. If, like us, you're a fan of baked desserts and apricots, this tart will not disappoint.

SERVES 8–10

FOR THE TART
1 x 320g sheet plant-based
    shortcrust pastry
6–8 apricots
3 tbsp apricot jam
1 tbsp water

FOR THE FRANGIPANE
75g plant-based butter,
    plus extra for greasing
100g caster sugar, plus
    25g for sprinkling
75g aquafaba (chickpea
    tin water)
1 tsp almond extract
1 tsp vanilla extract
50g plain flour
1 tbsp cornflour
180g ground almonds
½ tsp baking powder
pinch of sea salt

FOR THE CHANTILLY CREAM
320ml plant-based
    whipping cream
1½ tbsp icing sugar
1 tsp vanilla extract

Preheat oven to 180°C • 20cm tart tin • Baking paper • Baking beans or rice • Whisk • Small saucepan • Pastry brush • Sieve

Cook the pastry • Grease the tart tin with a little butter • Use the pastry to line the base and sides of the tart tin, cutting around the top to create neat edges • Prick the base with a fork then scrunch up a piece of baking paper and press into the case • Fill with baking beans or rice • Bake in the oven for 15 minutes • After 15 minutes, remove the beans or rice and the baking paper and bake for a further 10 minutes, until the pastry is lightly golden and dry to the touch

Make the frangipane • In a large mixing bowl, whisk the butter with the 100g caster sugar until pale • Gradually add the aquafaba, whisking with each addition • Add the almond and vanilla extracts • In a separate bowl, sift the flour together with the cornflour, ground almonds, baking powder and salt • Fold the dry mixture into the wet mixture until it comes together

Assemble the tart • Allow the tart case to cool to room temperature • Destone the apricots and cut the fruit into 1cm-thick slices • Once the pastry has cooled, sprinkle it with the remaining 25g sugar • Spoon the frangipane mixture into the tart case and use the back of the spoon to spread it evenly around • Top with the sliced apricots, placing them in a spiral pattern and pressing them into the frangipane • Bake in the oven for 35–45 minutes, until golden and the filling is set

Make the Chantilly cream • In the large mixing bowl, whip the cream to soft peaks • Add the icing sugar and vanilla extract and mix again to combine

Finish the tart • In a small saucepan, mix the apricot jam with the tablespoon of water and place over a low heat • Melt to a syrupy consistency • Once the tart is cooked, brush it with the apricot syrup and set aside to cool

Time to serve • Serve each slice of the tart with a few dollops of Chantilly cream

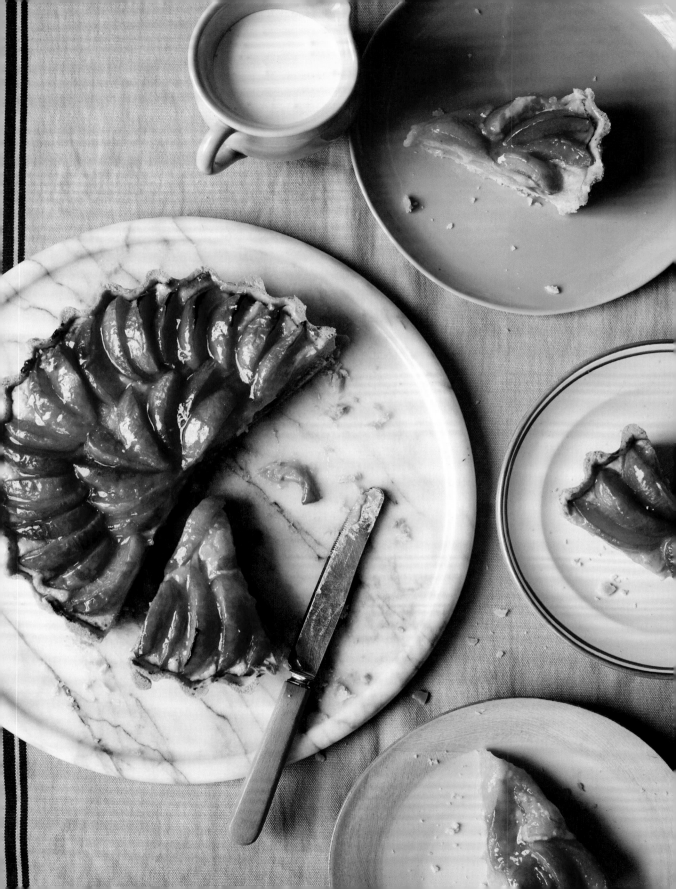

COFFEE AND WALNUT CAKE

Cake is good and coffee is good but when you put them both together, greatness happens. This recipe has the perfect balance of rich espresso coffee baked into a soft walnut sponge with bigger chunks of walnut for that extra crunch, sandwiched together with a coffee-infused buttercream icing. If you're like us and you enjoy a nice slice of cake every now and then, you simply need to make one of these because it might well be the best cake we've ever made. Yup, you read that right, the BEST cake we've ever made.

**MAKES 1 LARGE CAKE
(SERVES 12)**

FOR THE CAKE
2 tbsp apple cider vinegar
450ml oat milk
150g plant-based butter
    (block), plus extra
    for greasing
3 heaped tbsp instant
    espresso coffee powder
3 tbsp boiling water
400g light muscovado sugar
500g self-raising flour
2 tsp baking powder
½ tsp table salt
100g walnuts

FOR THE ICING
1 tbsp instant espresso
    coffee powder
½ tbsp boiling water
80g plant-based butter
450g icing sugar
2½ tbsp oat milk

FOR THE TOP
50g chopped walnuts

Preheat oven to 180°C • Small saucepan • Leave the plant-based butter for the icing out at room temperature • Grease 2 x 23cm cake tins and line the base and sides with baking parchment • Whisk • Wire rack • Spatula

Prepare the ingredients for the cake • Mix together the apple cider vinegar and oat milk in a small bowl and set aside for at least 15 minutes, until needed • Melt the butter in a small saucepan over a medium heat • Once melted, leave to cool to room temperature before making the cake

Make the cake • Put the instant coffee powder in a small bowl and add the boiling water • Mix well until the mixture comes together and becomes smooth • Spoon the sugar, flour, baking powder and salt into a large bowl and mix well until there are no lumps • Roughly chop the walnuts and mix them through the flour mixture • Pour the cooled butter, oat milk and coffee mixture into the bowl and mix well until a thick, smooth batter forms • Divide the batter evenly between 2 lined cake tins and bake in the oven for 30 minutes, or until the cake is cooked through (a knife inserted into the middle of each cake should come out clean – if not, place back in the oven for another 5–10 minutes)

Make the icing • Mix the instant coffee powder with the boiling water in a bowl until it has dissolved, then leave to cool • Place the room-temperature butter, icing sugar, oat milk and cooled coffee mixture into a large bowl and whisk until smooth

Cool the cakes • Once the cakes are cooked, remove from the oven and leave to cool for a few minutes then flip onto a wire rack • Leave to cool completely until they reach room temperature

Ice the cake • Place one cake onto a serving plate and top with half of the icing • Use a spatula to spread the icing out over the cake evenly • Top with the other cake before finishing with the remaining icing on top • Use a spatula to spread the icing out over the cake evenly before topping the cake with the chopped walnuts

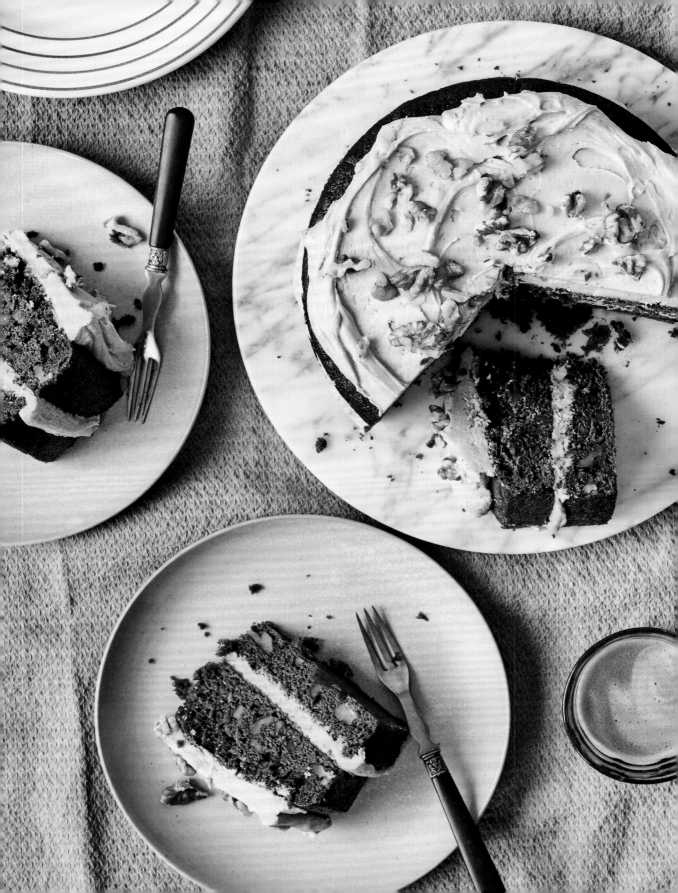

CREME BRÛLÉE

Sweet dreams are made of crème brûlée, who am I to disagree? I travelled the world and the seven seas, everybody's looking for something. If you're looking for 'something' – and if the 'something' you're looking for is creamy and sweet, with a delicious, crispy top – look no further, you've found it. The creamy set base is flavoured with vanilla and sugar for the perfect sweet treat, topped with a layer of caramelised sugar to crack your way through with that satisfying crunch. You can get ahead and make it the day before, and just give it a good go-over with the blowtorch just before serving.

SERVES 4

FOR THE BASE
150g raw unsalted cashews
1 x 300g pack silken tofu
2 tsp good-quality vanilla
    extract
70g golden caster sugar
70ml water

FOR THE TOPPING
4 tbsp golden caster sugar

Kettle boiled • Powerful blender • Small saucepan • 4 small ramekins • Deep baking tray • Blowtorch

Prepare the cashews • Put the cashews in a heatproof bowl and cover with boiling water • Set aside for at least 2 hours until needed

Make the base • After 2 hours, drain the cashews and place into a powerful blender • Drain the silken tofu and add it to the blender with the vanilla extract • Blend until really smooth and creamy • Preheat oven to 160°C

Make the sugar syrup • Place the sugar and water into a small saucepan over a low heat and cook, swirling the pan occasionally (not stirring) for 10 minutes or until all of the sugar granules have dissolved • Quickly pour the sugar syrup into the blender and blend again to mix the sugar syrup through the mixture

Cook the creme brûlées • Spoon the mixture evenly into 4 small ramekins and place into a deep baking tray • Boil the kettle and pour boiling water into the baking tray (around the ramekin bottoms, ensuring not to reach the top of them) • Cook in the oven for 15 minutes until set with a slight wobble

Chill the creme brûlées • After 10 minutes, remove the ramekins from the oven and leave to cool before placing in the fridge to firm up overnight

Finish the creme brûlées • Shortly before serving, sprinkle each ramekin with 1 tablespoon of sugar and blowtorch to caramelise

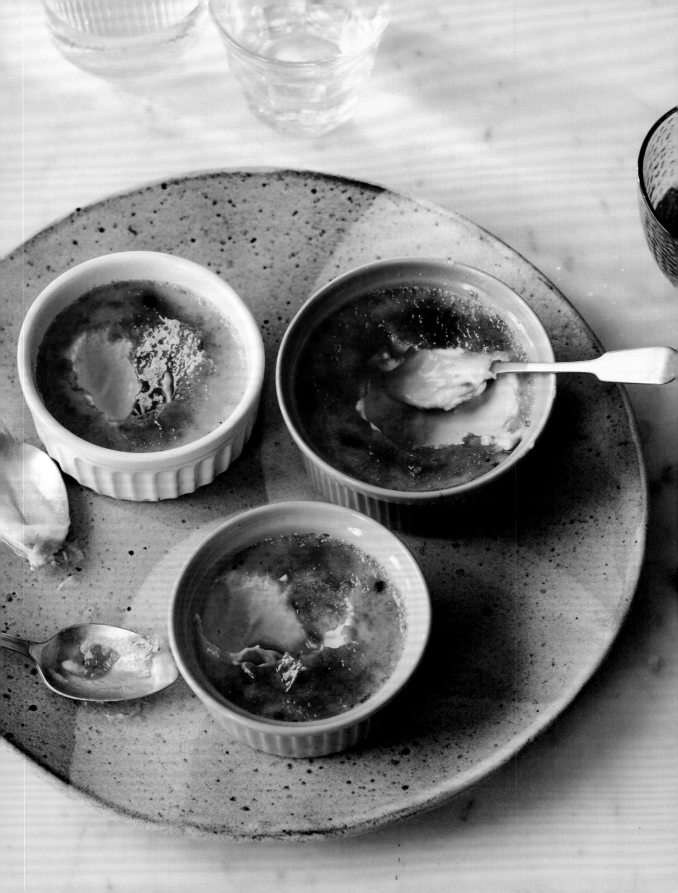

ETON MESS

This bonafide British classic proves that delicious desserts don't have to be stodgy and heavy to be satisfying. Perfectly sweet, curiously crispy and bursting with juicy fruit, this is the perfect dessert for a bright sunshiny day. Crunchy plant-based meringue is layered with fruity homemade berry purée, mixed with plant-based cream and topped with fresh mint. One of the best things about this dessert is that it's impossible to make it look bad!

SERVES 8

FOR THE MERINGUES
170g aquafaba (chickpea tin
    water)
1 tsp cream of tartar
150g caster sugar

FOR THE FRUIT PURÉE
100g strawberries
100g raspberries
30g icing sugar

**FOR THE CHANTILLY
CREAM**
450ml plant-based
    whipping cream
2 tbsp icing sugar

TO SERVE
200g strawberries
100g raspberries
fresh mint leaves

Preheat oven to 100°C • Electric whisk • 2 baking sheets lined with baking paper • Powerful blender

Make the meringues • Tip the aquafaba into a large mixing bowl and use an electric whisk to beat for 7–10 minutes, until thick and the mixture is aerated and forms soft peaks • Add the cream of tartar, then the sugar, a spoonful at a time, until the mixture is thick and glossy • Spoon the mixture onto the lined baking sheets in 8 big dollops (about 2 tablespoons per meringue) • Bake in the oven for 1 hour 45 minutes–2 hours, or until they come off the paper cleanly • Turn off the oven and leave them to cool completely in the oven – if you find the air is humid and they start to go sticky, continue cooking on low heat in the oven, or cook in the oven's residual heat until they become crisp again

Make the fruit purée • Remove the green tops from the strawberries • Put the strawberries and raspberries in a powerful blender along with the icing sugar • Blend to a purée

Make the Chantilly cream • In a large mixing bowl, whip the cream to soft peaks • Add the icing sugar and mix again to combine

Time to serve • Remove the green tops from the strawberries and slice • Roughly crush the meringues and stir three-quarters of them through the cream, along with most of the chopped strawberries and whole raspberries • Fold in the fruit purée to create a marble effect • Spoon into bowls, top with the remaining meringues (roughly crushed), chopped fruit and mint leaves • If you prefer, you can build the messes in individual glasses

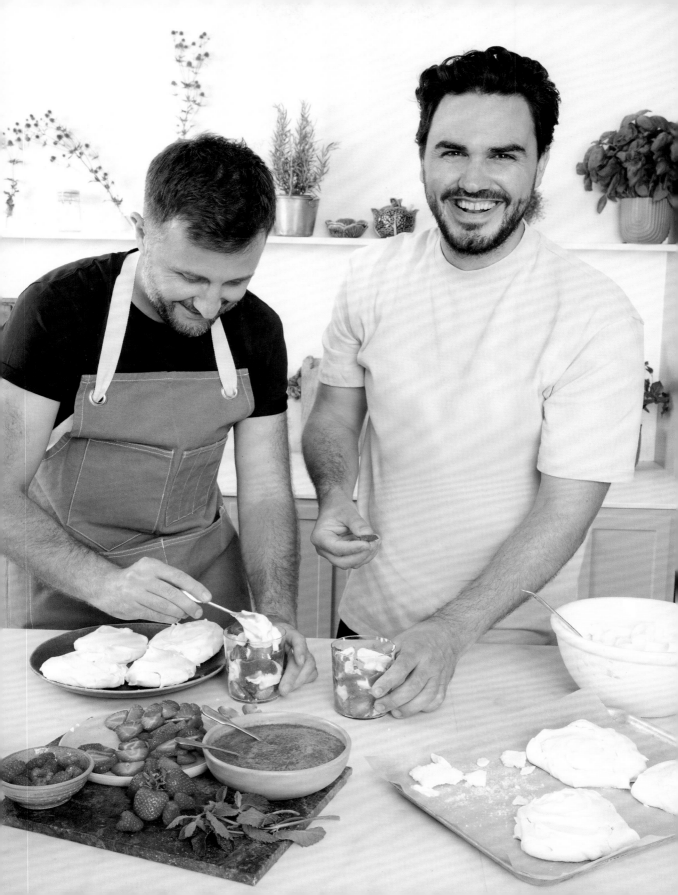

ECCLESALL ECCLES CAKES

Ian grew up in an area of Sheffield called Ecclesall and, on the walk home from school, he'd sometimes pop into the local bakery and treat himself to an Eccles cake: crispy, crunchy, kinda crumbly and bursting with juicy raisins. Eccles cakes are a delightful sweet treat and, if you've never tried them before, we urge you to make a batch. Serve with a chunk of plant-based cheddar if you're feeling frisky!

SERVES 8

FOR THE FILLING
30g dried apricots
15g plant-based butter
1 orange
1 tsp cornflour
60g dark brown sugar
85g currants and sultanas
   (use a mixture)
30g mixed candied peel
½ tsp ground allspice

FOR THE PASTRY
1 x 320g ready-rolled
   plant-based puff
   pastry sheet
oat milk, to glaze
3 tbsp demerara sugar

TO SERVE (OPTIONAL)
plant-based cheese, to
   serve (we like mature
   cheddar)

Fine grater or microplane • 10cm cookie cutter • Baking sheet lined with baking paper • Pastry brush

Make the filling • Chop the dried apricots and butter into small pieces and place into a mixing bowl • Grate in the zest from the orange, halve the orange and squeeze in 1 tablespoon of juice • Add the rest of the filling ingredients and mix until well combined

Shape the pastry • Unroll the pastry sheet • Use a 10cm cookie cutter to cut 8 round circles – you might need to collect the scraps and use them to make 8

Assemble the Eccles cakes • Place a heaped tablespoon of the fruit filling into the middle of a pastry circle • Brush around the edges with oat milk • Use your hands to draw the pastry up around and over the filling, giving it a good pinch together so the filling is all encased • Flip over and press the pastry flat • Use a knife to cut 2 slices in the top • Once assembled, transfer each cake to a baking sheet lined with baking paper • Repeat with the remaining circles • Once all of the cakes are made, place them in the fridge for 30 minutes to firm up • Preheat oven to 180°C

Bake the cakes • Brush each cake with oat milk and sprinkle with the demerara sugar • Bake in the oven for 20–30 minutes, until golden brown and crisp

Time to serve • Serve the cakes on a platter with wedges of plant-based cheese (if using)

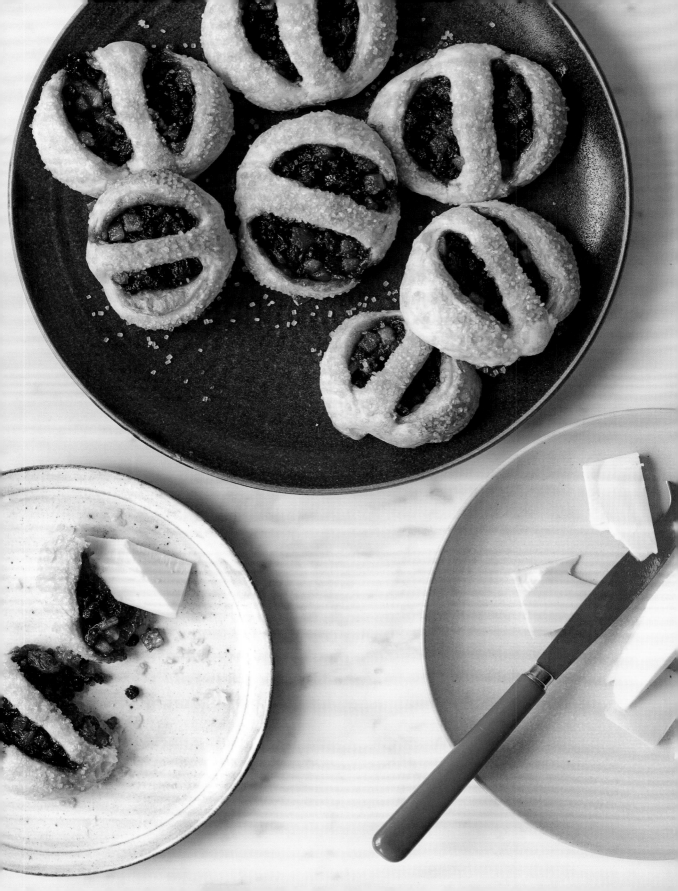

RED VELVET CAKE

If you've followed us for a while you probably know we LOVE cake. In fact, we love cakes so much we started selling them in UK supermarkets! We've done chocolate, lemon, vanilla and carrot, but we haven't done a red velvet, which is why we've given you this scrumptious recipe. This cake is a real showstopper – we first made it three tiers high, with layers of the cream cheese frosting sandwiching it together (and a few toothpicks!). The sponge is soft and bright red in colour with a super creamy vanilla frosting: everyone will love it!

**MAKES 1 LARGE CAKE
(SERVES 12)**

FOR THE CAKE
2 tbsp apple cider vinegar
450ml oat milk
150g plant-based
    butter (block), plus
    extra for greasing
400g golden caster sugar
500g self-raising flour
2 tsp baking powder
1 tbsp cacao powder
½ tsp table salt
½–1 tsp plant-based red
    food colouring

**FOR THE CREAM
CHEESE FROSTING**
100g plant-based butter
500g icing sugar
125g plant-based cream
    cheese
1 tsp vanilla extract

FOR THE TOP
10g freeze-dried
    raspberries or a handful
    of fresh strawberries

Preheat oven to 180°C • Grease 2 x 20cm cake tins and line the base and sides with baking parchment • Leave the plant-based butter for the frosting out at room temperature • Small saucepan • Food processor • Wire rack • Spatula

Prepare the ingredients • Mix together the vinegar and oat milk in a small bowl and set aside until needed • Melt the butter in a small saucepan • Once melted, leave to cool before making the cake

Make the cake batter • Spoon the sugar, flour, baking powder, cacao and salt into a large bowl and mix well until there are no lumps • Pour in the cooled butter and oat milk and mix well until a thick, smooth batter forms

Colour the cake batter • Add ½ teaspoon of the red food colouring and mix it through the batter – if the colour is not a really bright and vivid red, add another ½ teaspoon and mix through

Bake the cakes • Divide the batter evenly between 2 lined cake tins and bake in the oven for 30 minutes, or until the cakes are cooked through (a knife inserted into the middle of each cake should come out clean - if not, place back in the oven for another 5–10 minutes)

Make the frosting • Put the room-temperature butter, icing sugar, cream cheese and vanilla extract in a food processor and blend until smooth

Cool the cakes • Once the cakes are cooked, remove from the oven and leave to sit in the tins for a few minutes, then flip them onto a wire rack and remove the baking parchment • Leave to cool completely until room temperature

Ice the cake • Place one cake half onto a serving plate and top with half of the frosting • Use a spatula to spread the frosting out over the cake evenly • Top with the other cake before adding the rest of the frosting • Use a spatula to spread the frosting out over the cake evenly

For the top • If using freeze-dried raspberries, crush the freeze-dried raspberries and sprinkle around the edges of the top of the cake • If using fresh strawberries, cut the strawberries in half and place the halves around the top of the cake (if using fresh strawberries, serve the cake immediately so they remain in place)

NOTE
You can make this cake with 3 tiers for an extra-impressive centrepiece • Simply divide the batter equally between 3 x 20cm cake tins and bake for 30 minutes • When assembling the cake, divide the frosting in thirds between the cake layers • As the cake is so large with three tiers, you can use cake dowels to hold it together

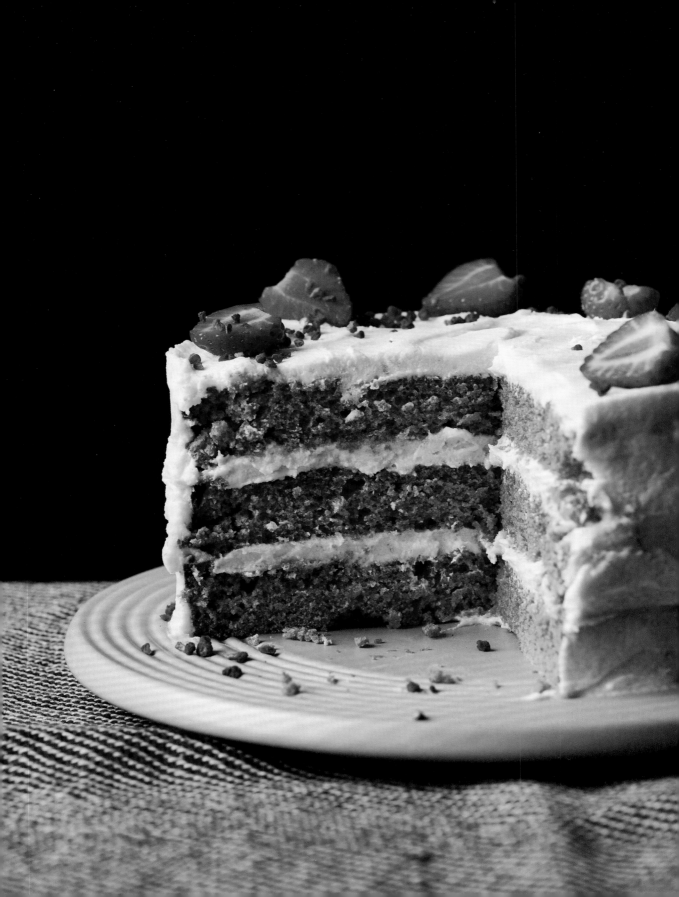

STRAYA LAMINGTONS

Lamingtons are one of Australia's favourite sweet treats and we certainly see why. Soft sponge cake sandwiched together with sweet raspberry jam, coated in a layer of dark chocolate sauce and sprinkled with coconut – what could be better?

MAKES 6

FOR THE SPONGE
1 tbsp cider vinegar
225ml oat milk
80g plant-based
    butter (block), plus
    extra for greasing
200g caster sugar
250g self-raising flour
1 tsp baking powder
½ tsp table salt

FOR THE CHOCOLATE SAUCE
200g dark chocolate
50g plant-based butter
100ml oat milk
200g icing sugar
50g cacao powder

FOR THE MIDDLE
1 jar of raspberry jam

FOR THE TOPPING
desiccated coconut, to coat

Small saucepan • Large baking tray (about 20 x 30 x 3cm) lined with baking parchment • Wire rack • Sieve

Prepare the ingredients for the sponge • Mix together the cider vinegar and oat milk in a small bowl and leave to one side for at least 20 minutes • Melt the butter in a small saucepan over a medium heat • Once completely melted, leave to cool to room temperature before making the cake • Preheat oven to 180°C

Make the sponge • Spoon the sugar, flour, baking powder and salt into a large bowl and mix well until there are no lumps • Pour the cooled butter and the oat milk mixture into the bowl and mix well until a thick, smooth batter forms • Pour the batter into a lined baking tray and bake in the oven for 25–30 minutes, or until the sponge is cooked through (a knife inserted in the middle should come out clean – if not, place back in the oven for another 5–10 minutes)

Cool the sponge • Once the sponge has cooked, remove from the oven and flip onto a wire rack • Leave to cool completely until room temperature

Make the sauce • Break the chocolate into pieces • Put the chocolate and butter in a small saucepan over a very low heat and cook for a few minutes, constantly stirring until the chocolate starts to melt • Once the chocolate begins to melt, add the oat milk and mix well over the heat until all of the chocolate has melted • Once the chocolate has melted, sift in the icing sugar and cacao powder • Mix well and cook for 3–5 minutes until the sauce comes together to create a smooth consistency • Turn off the heat and leave to cool a little

Make the lamingtons • Sprinkle plenty of desiccated coconut into a baking tray • Cut two lines lengthways down the middle of the cooled sponge, before cutting 3 lines widthways – this should leave you with 12 equal cube shapes • Spread the jam on one side of one of the cake cubes and place another cake cube on top, like a jam sandwich (you can neaten up with a knife around the edges if needed) • Place them on a wire rack set over a baking tray and spoon over the chocolate sauce to completely and evenly cover them, then – working quickly – place them in the coconut and coat before returning them to the wire rack • Stored in an airtight container in the fridge or a chilled space, they'll last a couple of days

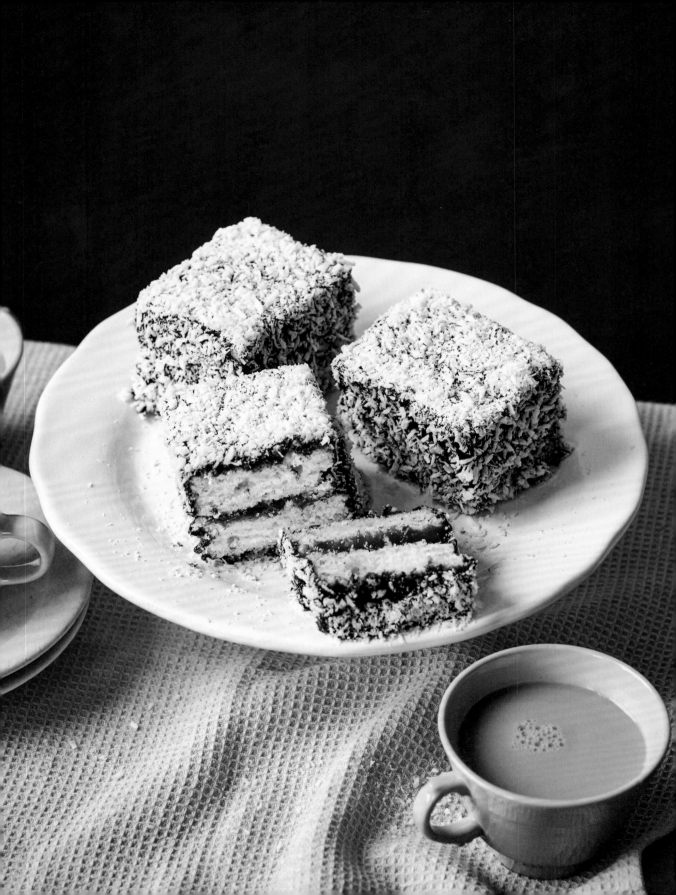

SHEET-PAN SHARING PANCAKE

Pancakes can be frustrating because they come out of the pan at different times. A family will either eat their pancakes individually, when they're nice and hot, or together as a group, when some of the pancakes are cold and soggy. It's a problem! Our Sheet-pan Sharing Pancake solves this problem by enabling families to eat hot, delicious slices of fluffy pancake around the kitchen table together. Pour the pancake batter onto a large baking tray, drizzle with runny nut butter, and swirl it through for a beautiful marbled look that everyone will love. It's great served with plant-based cream, maple syrup, mugs of tea and people you care about.

SERVES 6

FOR THE PANCAKE
350g self-raising flour
3 tbsp caster sugar
1 tsp baking powder
¼ tsp table salt
400ml almond milk
2 tbsp vegetable oil

FOR THE TOPPING
1 jar of runny almond
   or peanut butter
   (about 150g)
handful of raspberries (or
   any fruit of your choice),
   plus extra to serve

TO SERVE
maple syrup
plant-based cream

Preheat oven to 180°C • Large baking tray lined with baking paper

Make the pancake batter • Put the flour, sugar, baking powder and salt in a large mixing bowl and whisk until there are no lumps • Pour in the almond milk and vegetable oil and whisk again until the mixture forms a smooth batter

Cook the pancake • Pour the batter into the lined baking tray • Drizzle some nut butter over the top and use a teaspoon to create a marble-like consistency over the top of the batter • Sprinkle with the raspberries (or whatever fruit you are using) • Bake the pancake in the oven for 15–20 minutes, or until golden and cooked through

Time to serve • Serve the pancake while hot with a side of fresh berries, maple syrup and plant-based cream

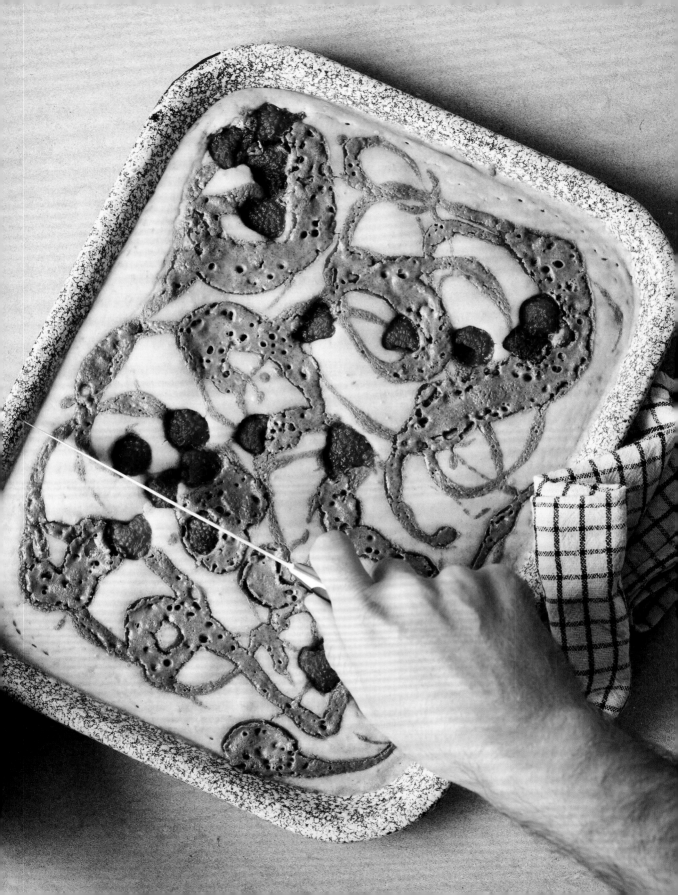

MILLE-FEUILLE

Creamy thick custard and crispy sweet pastry combine to form a truly delectable dessert that looks as good as it tastes. This one took a little while to perfect but, by jove, the time it took was absolutely worth it. Make a batch next time your nan's coming over; she'll be chuffed.

SERVES 9

FOR THE PASTRY
2 x 320g ready-rolled
    plant-based puff pastry
sheets

FOR THE CUSTARD FILLING
100g caster sugar
100g plant-based custard
    powder
4 tbsp cornflour
800ml oat milk
100ml plant-based cream
1 tsp vanilla extract

TO SERVE
icing sugar

Preheat oven to 180°C • 2 baking trays • Whisk • Heavy-based saucepan • Piping bag

Bake the pastry • Unroll a sheet of pastry onto a baking tray, leaving it on the paper it comes with • Cover with a sheet of baking paper, then top with another baking tray • Top with something ovenproof and heavy – we use a casserole dish • Place in the oven and cook for 30–35 minutes until the pastry turns golden brown

Meanwhile, make the custard • Put the sugar, custard powder and cornflour in a large mixing bowl and mix until there are no lumps • Gradually whisk in the oat milk to avoid any lumps • Once the milk has been mixed in, add the cream and vanilla extract and mix again until everything is well combined • Pour the mixture into a heavy-based saucepan and place over a low heat • Cook until very thick, whisking regularly to avoid any lumps forming • Once the mixture has thickened, spoon it back into a heatproof mixing bowl and cover with cling film • Leave to cool then transfer to the fridge to set for at least 2 hours

Finish the pastry sheets • Once the pastry sheet is cooked, set it aside and repeat the process with the remaining sheet of pastry • Once cooked, set the pastry aside to cool

Prepare the custard • Once the custard has set firm, remove it from the fridge and whisk again to loosen up the mixture and ensure there are no lumps • Spoon the custard into a piping bag – if you don't have a piping bag, you can just spread the custard between the sheets of pastry using a spoon

Assemble the mille-feuille • Once the pastry sheets have cooled, cut them into 18 rectangles (about 3 x 10cm) • Lay out a rectangle of pastry, then either pipe or spread the custard filling on top • Place another sheet of pastry over the top and dust with icing sugar

Time to serve • Place the mille-feuilles in the fridge until needed (up to 2 days) – this will also allow the custard to set in shape

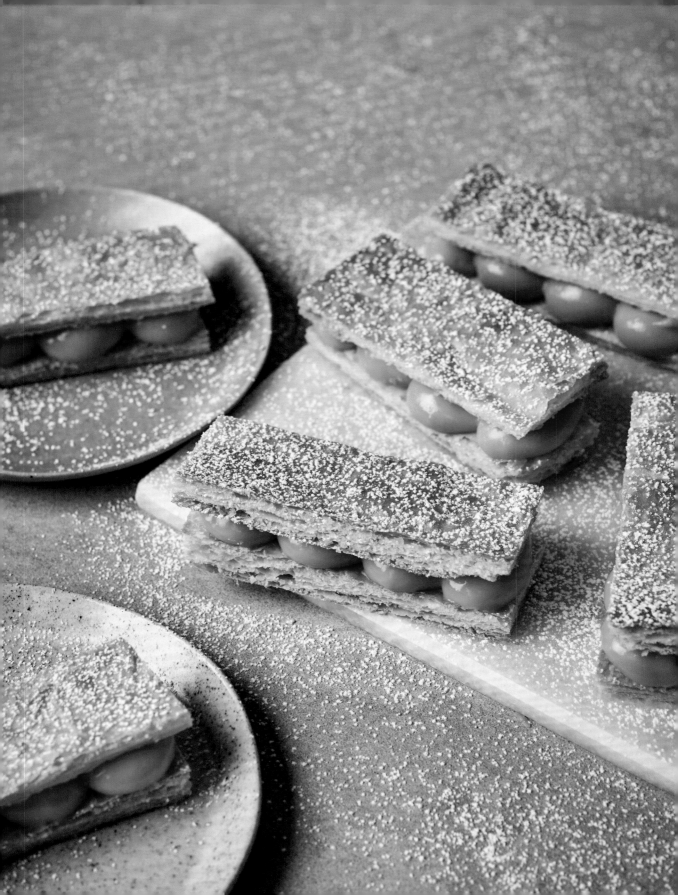

PRETTY PALMIERS

These lovely little things remind us of the decorations found on ancient Greek terracotta pottery. They also remind us how satisfying it is to bake tasty treats at home. Easy, tasty and perfect with a cup of tea – what's not to like?

MAKES 16

1 x 320g ready-rolled plant-based puff pastry sheet
90g sugar (we use a mix of caster sugar, granulated sugar and soft light brown sugar)
1 tsp ground cinnamon (optional)

2 baking trays lined with baking paper

Prepare the pastry • Unroll the puff pastry sheet so the shortest edge is facing you, keeping the pastry paper on the base • Mix the sugars together with the cinnamon (if using) • Scatter three-quarters of the sugar over the pastry sheet

Shape the palmiers • Fold the left and the right sides in to meet in the middle • Scatter with the remaining sugar • Wrap the roll with the pastry paper around it – squeezing the roll so that the pastry stays together, otherwise it will unravel – then wrap in cling film • Place in the fridge for 45 minutes to firm up • Preheat oven to 200°C

Bake the palmiers • Use a large serrated knife to cut the log into 16 x 1cm-thick slices • Place the slices face down on a baking tray lined with baking paper, 5cm apart from each other • Bake in the oven for 15–20 minutes, until caramelised and golden • Allow to cool before serving

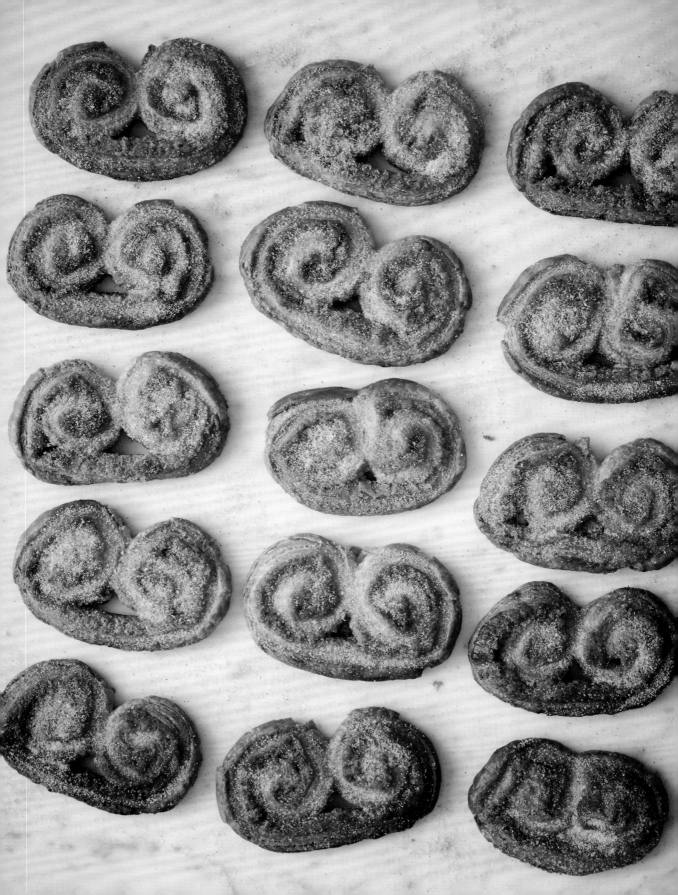

INDEX

A

almond milk: bacon cauliflower cheese 202
creamy red pepper penne 48
sheet-pan sharing pancake 240
almonds: apricot tart 226
apple gravy 118–19
apricots: apricot tart 226
spicy apricot, chickpea and lamb tagine 164–5
aquafaba (chickpea tin water): Eton mess 232
asparagus: date-night scallops 174
seafood paella 194
aubergines (eggplant): cheesy chicken enchiladas and Mexican-style corn salad 50–1
iskender kebab with spiced tomato sauce 146–7
avocados: 80s prawn cocktail 170
guacamole 88–9

B

bacon 29
bacon cauliflower cheese 202
bacon fishcakes with minty pea mash and lemon hollandaise sauce 188
bacon sprouts 105
boeuf bourguignon 92
mushroom bacon 74

ultimate Bolognese 81
Baja fish tacos 196–7
banana blossom: moqueca 176
seafood paella 194
basil: pesto 57
BBQ sauce: BBQ smash burgers 98
rack o' ribs 130
beansprouts: blackened monk chicken noodles 54
pho king 114
Thai salad 65
beef 32, 76–107
BBQ smash burgers 98
boeuf bourguignon 92
carne asada tacos 88–9
chilli cheeseburger nachos 82
crispy shredded beef with egg-fried rice 100
keema paratha with coconut chutney 86
Lancashire hotpot 150
orzo meatballs 84
Philly cheesesteak 78
quattro formaggi lasagne 210
South African bobotie 94–5
ultimate Bolognese 81
Wellington 102–3
bhuna: meaty bhuna and aromatic pilau rice 158–9
big Bosh meaty Sunday lunch 102–5
binders 18
biscotti biscuits: tiramisu 224

black beans: blackened monk chicken noodles 54
bobotie, South African 94–5
boeuf bourguignon 92
Bolognese, ultimate 81
borlotti beans: Tuscan tuna pasta salad 184
Brazilian fish stew 176
bread: Chippy's hottest dog 132
ko club sandwich 74
nigella naan 140–1
pesto chicken sandwich 57
prawn linguine and garlic ciabatta 190
shrimp po'boy 192
brioche buns: BBQ smash burgers 98
fillet – WOAH – fish 172
lobster roll 182
Philly cheesesteak 78
broad beans: minty pea mash 188
broccoli: blackened monk chicken noodles 54
Lancashire hotpot 150
broth: pho king 114
burger sauce 82
burgers, BBQ smash 98
butter 41
seaweed butter 174
butterbean mash 112

C

cabbage: curtido 196–7
pork gyoza with zippy dippy 122
Thai salad 65
cakes: coffee and

walnut cake 228
5-minute mug cake 222
red velvet cake 236
caramelised onion mash 118–19
carne asada tacos 88–9
carrots: boeuf bourguignon 92
carrot and daikon pickle 54
kare raisu 62
Lancashire hotpot 150
maple-roasted parsnips and carrots 104
South African bobotie 94–5
Thai salad 65
cashews: Cheddar 36
chilli cheeseburger nachos 82
creamy red pepper penne 48
crème brûlée 230
lemon hollandaise sauce 188
poutine 214
cauliflower cheese, bacon 202
Chantilly cream 226, 232
char sui pork 116
cheese 200–19
bacon cauliflower cheese 202
BBQ smash burgers 98
carne asada tacos 88–9
Cheddar 36
cheese and mushroom omelette 204
cheesy chicken enchiladas and Mexican-style corn salad 50–1

chilli cheeseburger
nachos 82
chorizo mac and
cheese 206
fillet – WOAH – fish 172
giant couscous and
feta salad 138
Greek salad 64–5
Philly cheesesteak 78
poutine 214
quattro formaggi
lasagne 210
sausage and stuffing
pastry puffs 134
sausage party pizza
216–17
silky polenta 144
spanakopita
with tomato and
pomegranate za'atar
salad 208
cheeseburger nachos,
chilli 82
cheesesteak, Philly 78
chestnuts: Wellington
102–3
chicken 30
blackened monk
chicken noodles 54
cheesy chicken
enchiladas and
Mexican-style
corn salad 50–1
chicken skewers
– 3 ways 64–5
chicken tikka
masala 68
Coronation chicken
salad 60
creamy red pepper
penne 48
crispy Korean-style
chicken wings 46
five-minute noodles 45
kare raisu 62
kung pao chicken 72

pesto chicken
sandwich 57
chickpeas: bacon 29
chicken 30
sausages 26
spicy apricot, chickpea
and lamb tagine with
saffron couscous
164–5
chillies: cheesy
chicken enchiladas
and Mexican-style
corn salad 50–1
chilli cheeseburger
nachos 82
chipotle mayo 196–7
Chippy's hottest dog 132
crispy Korean-style
chicken wings 46
guacamole 88–9
keema paratha with
coconut chutney 86
Chinese pancakes: duck
pancakes 70
Chippy's hottest dog 132
chips: poutine 214
chocolate: 5-minute
mug cake 222
red velvet cake 236
straya lamingtons 238
chorizo sausages:
chorizo bangers with
butterbean mash 112
chorizo mac and
cheese 206
chorizo risotto 126
chow-down
chowder 180
chutney, coconut 86
coconut: coconut
chutney 86
straya lamingtons 238
coconut milk:
Cheddar 36
gaeng phed ped yang
with coconut rice 58

moqueca 176
prawn malai 186
coconut oil: butter 41
coffee: coffee and
walnut cake 228
tiramisu 224
colourings, natural 18
Coronation chicken
salad 60
couscous: giant
couscous and feta
salad 138
saffron couscous
164–5
cream, Chantilly
226, 232
cream cheese: creamy
cheese frosting 236
tiramisu 224
crème brûlée 230
crème fraîche: creamy
leeks 105
crispy Korean-style
chicken wings 46
crispy shredded beef
with egg-fried rice 100
cucumber: duck
pancakes 70
easy tzatziki 156
Greek salad 64–5
kachumber 186
teriyaki skewers with
cucumber salad 64
curry: chicken tikka
masala 68
Coronation chicken
salad 60
gaeng phed ped yang
with coconut rice 58
kare raisu 62
Kashmiri lamb with
dum aloo and nigella
naan 140–1
meaty bhuna and
aromatic pilau rice
158–9

prawn malai 186
South African
bobotie 94–5
custard: mille-feuille 242

D
daikon: carrot and
daikon pickle 54
date-night scallops 174
dates: harissa-spiced
pulled lamb with giant
couscous and feta
salad 138
dips: dipping sauces
122, 130
garlic and herb dip
216–17
dried fruit: Ecclesall
Eccles cakes 234
see also raisins
duck: duck pancakes 70
gaeng phed ped yang
with coconut rice 58
dum aloo 140–1

E
Ecclesall Eccles cakes 234
eggs: crispy shredded
beef with egg-fried
rice 100
80s prawn cocktail 170
enchiladas, cheesy
chicken 50–1
Eton mess 232

F
fats 18
fennel: ultimate
Bolognese 81
fillers 19
filo pastry:
spanakopita 208
fish: bacon fishcakes
with minty pea
mash and lemon
hollandaise sauce 188

baked tuna puttanesca
with crispy
gnocchi 178
fillet – WOAH – fish 172
fish (tuna) 35
moqueca 176
Tuscan tuna pasta
salad 184
5-minute mug cake 222
five-minute noodles 45
flatbreads, Lebanese-
style lamb 162
flavourings, natural 18
frangipane: apricot tart
226
fries 172
frosting, creamy cheese
236
fruit: Eton mess 232

G
gaeng phed ped yang
with coconut rice 58
garlic: chicken tikka
masala 68
crispy Korean-style
chicken wings 46
dum aloo 140–1
garlic and herb dip
216–17
prawn linguine and
garlic ciabatta 190
ultimate Bolognese 81
gnocchi, baked tuna
puttanesca with crispy
178
gravy 104, 112, 214
apple gravy 118–19
whisky gravy 152–3
Greek salad 64–5
Greek stuffed peppers
156
green beans: seafood
paella 194
greens 16
guacamole 88–9

gyoza, pork 122

H
haggis, neeps and
tatties with whisky
gravy 152–3
halloumi: hearty
halloumi salad 212
harissa-spiced
pulled lamb with giant
couscous and feta
salad 138
hearts of palm: lobster
roll 182
herbs: garlic and herb
dip 216–17
hollandaise sauce,
lemon 188
hot dogs: Chippy's
hottest dog 132
hotpot, Lancashire 150

I
iskender kebab with
spiced tomato sauce
146–7

J
jackfruit: beef 32
cheesy chicken
enchiladas and
Mexican-style corn
salad 50–1
duck pancakes 70
harissa-spiced
pulled lamb with giant
couscous and feta
salad 138
iskender kebab with
spiced tomato sauce
146–7
Kashmiri lamb with
dum aloo and nigella
naan 140–1
Lancashire hotpot 150
luscious lamb ragu with

silky polenta 144
spicy apricot, chickpea
and lamb tagine with
saffron couscous
164–5

K
kachumber 186
kale, wilted 118–19
kare raisu 62
Kashmiri lamb with dum
aloo and nigella naan
140–1
kebabs: iskender kebab
with spiced tomato
sauce 146–7
keema paratha with
coconut chutney 86
kidney beans: haggis,
neeps and tatties
with whisky
gravy 152–3
ko club sandwich 74
Korean-style chicken
wings 46
kung pao chicken 72

L
labels, reading 17
lamb 136–67
harissa-spiced
pulled lamb with giant
couscous and feta
salad 138
iskender kebab with
spiced tomato sauce
146–7
Kashmiri lamb with
dum aloo and nigella
naan 140–1
Lancashire hotpot 150
Lebanese-style lamb
flatbreads with minty
yoghurt 162
luscious lamb ragu with
silky polenta 144

meaty bhuna and
aromatic pilau
rice 158–9
spicy apricot, chickpea
and lamb tagine with
saffron couscous
164–5
yemista with easy
tzatziki 156
Lancashire hotpot 150
lasagne, quattro
formaggi 210
Lebanese-style lamb
flatbreads with minty
yoghurt 162
leeks, creamy 105
lemon hollandaise sauce
188
lentils: Chippy's hottest
dog 132
South African bobotie
94–5
lettuce: BBQ smash
burgers 98
chilli cheeseburger
nachos 82
Coronation chicken
salad 60
80s prawn cocktail 170
ko club sandwich 74
lobster roll 182
Mexican-style corn
salad 50–1
linguine: prawn linguine
and garlic ciabatta 190
lobster roll 182
luscious lamb ragu with
silky polenta 144

M
mac and cheese,
chorizo 206
malai, prawn 186
maple-roasted parsnips
and carrots 104
Marie rose sauce 170

mash: butterbean
mash 112
caramelised onion
mash 118–19
minty pea mash 188
mayo, chipotle 196–7
meatballs, orzo 84
meaty bhuna and
aromatic pilau rice 158–9
menu planning 22–3
meringues: Eton mess 232
Mexican-style corn
salad 50–1
milk 38
mille-feuille 242
minerals 20
mint: mint yoghurt
138, 162
minty pea mash 188
minty rocket and
kalamata salad 156
moqueca 176
mug cake, 5-minute 222
mushrooms: boeuf
bourguignon 92
cheese and mushroom
omelette 204
Coronation chicken
salad 60
date-night scallops 174
haggis, neeps and
tatties with whisky
gravy 152–3
harissa-spiced pulled
lamb with giant
couscous and feta
salad 138
ko club sandwich 74
luscious lamb ragu with
silky polenta 144
mushroom bacon 74
Philly cheesesteak 78
quattro formaggi
lasagne 210
rack o' ribs 130
seafood paella 194

ultimate Bolognese 81
weeping tiger jay 124
Wellington 102–3
yemista with easy
tzatziki 156

N
naan, nigella 140–1
nachos, chilli
cheeseburger 82
neeps and tatties,
haggis, 152–3
nigella naan 140–1
nooch (nutritional
yeast): Cheddar 36
creamy red pepper
penne 48
orzo meatballs 84
noodles: blackened
monk chicken
noodles 54
five-minute noodles 45
pho king 114
nutrients 20

O
oat milk 38
mille-feuille 242
olives: baked tuna
puttanesca with crispy
gnocchi 178
Greek salad 64–5
minty rocket and
kalamata salad 156
omelette, cheese and
mushroom 204
onions: boeuf
bourguignon 92
caramelised onion
mash 118–19
orzo meatballs 84

P
paella, seafood 194
pak choi: char sui
pork 116

palmiers, pretty 244
pancakes: duck
pancakes 70
sheet-pan sharing
pancake 240
paratha, keema 86
parsnips, maple-roasted
carrots and 104
pasta: chorizo mac and
cheese 206
creamy red pepper
penne 48
orzo meatballs 84
prawn linguine and
garlic ciabatta 190
quattro formaggi
lasagne 210
Sarah's succulent
sausage pasta 128
Tuscan tuna pasta
salad 184
pastry puffs, sausage
and stuffing 134
pea protein: beef 32
peanut butter: satay
skewers with Thai
salad 65
sheet-pan sharing
pancake 240
peanuts: kung pao
chicken 72
pearl barley: hearty
halloumi salad 212
peas: creamy leeks 105
crispy shredded beef
with egg-fried
rice 100
Lancashire hotpot 150
minty pea mash 188
peppers: cheesy
chicken enchiladas
and Mexican-style
corn salad 50–1
chorizo bangers
with butterbean
mash 112

creamy red pepper
penne 48
Greek stuffed peppers
156
hearty halloumi salad
212
kung pao chicken 72
Philly cheesesteak 78
pesto: pesto chicken
sandwich 57
Sarah's succulent
sausage pasta 128
petits pois: keema
paratha with coconut
chutney 86
Philly cheesesteak 78
pho king 114
pickle, carrot
and daikon 54
pico de gallo 196–7
pillowy pork
steamed buns 110
pine nuts: pesto 57
pittas: iskender kebab
with spiced tomato
sauce 146–7
pizza, sausage
party 216–17
plant meat, history
of 13
plates, mixing up your 16
plum sauce: duck
pancakes 70
po'boy, shrimp 192
polenta, luscious lamb
ragu with silky 144
pomegranate: giant
couscous and feta
salad 138
tomato and
pomegranate za'atar
salad 208
pork 108–35
char sui pork 116
Chippy's hottest dog
132

chorizo mac and
  cheese 206
chorizo risotto 126
pho king 114
pillowy pork steamed
  buns 110
pork belly and
  crackling with
  caramelised onion
  mash and apple gravy
  118–19
pork gyoza with zippy
  dippy 122
Sarah's succulent
  sausage pasta 128
sausage and stuffing
  pastry puffs 134
weeping tiger jay 124
potatoes: bacon
  fishcakes with minty
  pea mash 188
  boeuf bourguignon 92
  caramelised onion
  mash 118–19
  chilli cheeseburger
  nachos 82
  chow-down chowder 180
  dum aloo 140–1
  fries 172
  haggis, neeps and
  tatties with whisky
  gravy 152–3
  Lancashire hotpot 150
  poutine 214
  roast potatoes 103
poultry 42–75
  see also chicken; duck
poutine 214
prawns: 80s prawn
  cocktail 170
  moqueca 176
  prawn linguine and
  garlic ciabatta 190
  prawn malai 186
  seafood paella 194
  shrimp po'boy 192

preservatives 19
pretty palmiers 244
protein 18, 21
puff pastry: Ecclesall
  Eccles cakes 234
  mille-feuille 242
  pretty palmiers 244
  sausage and stuffing
  pastry puffs 134
  Wellington 102–3
puttanesca, baked
  tuna 178

Q
quattro formaggi
  lasagne 210

R
rack o' ribs 130
ragu: luscious lamb ragu
  with silky polenta 144
rainbow ratio 16
raisins: South African
  bobotie 94–5
  yemista with easy
  tzatziki 156
raspberries: Eton mess
  232
  sheet-pan sharing
  pancake 240
raspberry jam: straya
  lamingtons 238
red velvet cake 236
remoulade 192
rice: char sui pork 116
  chicken tikka masala 68
  chorizo risotto 126
  coconut rice 58
  crispy shredded beef
  with egg-fried rice 100
  kare raisu 62
  kung pao chicken 72
  meaty bhuna and
  aromatic pilau
  rice 158–9
  moqueca 176

prawn malai 186
seafood paella 194
South African bobotie
  94–5
weeping tiger jay 124
yemista with easy
  tzatziki 156
risotto, chorizo 126
rocket: minty rocket and
  kalamata salad 156
rum: tiramisu 224

S
saffron couscous 164–5
salads: Coronation
  chicken salad 60
  Greek salad 64–5
  harissa-spiced
  pulled lamb with giant
  couscous and feta
  salad 138
  hearty halloumi salad
  212
  Mexican-style corn
  salad 50–1
  minty rocket and
  kalamata salad 156
  spanakopita
  with tomato and
  pomegranate za'atar
  salad 208
  teriyaki skewers with
  cucumber salad 64
  Tuscan tuna pasta
  salad 184
sandwiches: ko club
  sandwich 74
  lobster roll 182
  pesto chicken
  sandwich 57
  Philly cheesesteak 78
  shrimp po'boy 192
  Sarah's succulent
  sausage pasta 128
satay skewers with Thai
  salad 65

sauces: burger sauce 82
  cheese sauce 82
  lemon hollandaise
  sauce 188
sausages 26
  Chippy's hottest dog
  132
  chorizo bangers
  with butterbean
  mash 112
  chorizo mac and
  cheese 206
  chorizo risotto 126
  luscious lamb ragu with
  silky polenta 144
  Sarah's succulent
  sausage pasta 128
  sausage and stuffing
  pastry puffs 134
  sausage party pizza
  216–17
scallops, date-night 174
seafood 168–99
seaweed butter 174
sheet-pan sharing
  pancake 240
shiitake mushrooms:
  weeping tiger jay 124
shrimp po'boy 192
skewers: chicken
  skewers – 3 ways 64–5
soup: chow-down
  chowder 180
South African bobotie
  94–5
souvlaki skewers with
  Greek salad 64–5
soy: meaty bhuna and
  aromatic pilau
  rice 158–9
soy milk: butter 41
  chicken 30
soy sauce: fish (tuna) 35
spanakopita with tomato
  and pomegranate
  za'atar salad 208

spicy apricot, chickpea and lamb tagine with saffron couscous 164–5

spinach: creamy red pepper penne 48

spanakopita with tomato and pomegranate za'atar salad 208

spring greens: Lancashire hotpot 150

weeping tiger jay 124

sprouts, bacon 105

steamed buns, pillowy pork 110

stew: moqueca 176

strawberries: Eton mess 232

straya lamingtons 238

stuffing: sausage and stuffing pastry puffs 134

swede: haggis, neeps and tatties with whisky gravy 152–3

sweet potatoes: chilli cheeseburger nachos 82

sweetcorn: chow-down chowder 180

Mexican-style corn salad 50–1

T

tacos: Baja fish tacos 196–7

carne asada tacos 88–9

tagine, spicy apricot, chickpea and lamb 164–5

tahini yoghurt 146–7

tapioca starch: fish (tuna) 35

tartare sauce 172

tarts: apricot tart 226

spanakopita with tomato and pomegranate za'atar salad 208

tempeh: Lebanese-style lamb flatbreads with minty yoghurt 162

tenderstem broccoli: Lancashire hotpot 150

teriyaki skewers with cucumber salad 64

Thai salad, satay skewers with 65

tikka masala, chicken 68

tiramisu 224

tofu: Baja fish tacos 196–7

cheese and mushroom omelette 204

chow-down chowder 180

crackling 118–19

crème brûlée 230

crispy Korean-style chicken wings 46

crispy shredded beef with egg-fried rice 100

fillet – WOAH – fish 172

hearty halloumi salad 212

South African bobotie 94–5

spanakopita with tomato and pomegranate za'atar salad 208

tomatoes: baked tuna puttanesca with crispy gnocchi 178

BBQ smash burgers 98

cheese and mushroom omelette 204

cheesy chicken enchiladas and Mexican-style corn salad 50–1

chicken tikka masala 68

chilli cheeseburger nachos 82

Chippy's hottest dog 132

chorizo risotto 126

creamy red pepper penne 48

dum aloo 140–1

gaeng phed ped yang with coconut rice 58

Greek salad 64–5

hearty halloumi salad 212

iskender kebab with spiced tomato sauce 146–7

kachumber 186

ko club sandwich 74

meaty bhuna and aromatic pilau rice 158–9

moqueca 176

orzo meatballs 84

pico de gallo 196–7

quattro formaggi lasagne 210

Sarah's succulent sausage pasta 128

sausage party pizza 216–17

seafood paella 194

spanakopita with tomato and pomegranate za'atar salad 208

Tuscan tuna pasta salad 184

ultimate Bolognese 81

tortilla chips: chilli cheeseburger nachos 82

tortillas: Baja fish tacos 196–7

tuna 35

bacon fishcakes with minty pea mash and lemon hollandaise sauce 188

baked tuna puttanesca with crispy gnocchi 178

Tuscan tuna pasta salad 184

tzatziki 156

U

ultimate Bolognese 81

V

vegetables 16

vitamins 16, 20

W

walnuts: coffee and walnut cake 228

weeping tiger jay 124

Wellington 102–3

whisky gravy 152–3

wine: boeuf bourguignon 92

gravy 104, 214

kare raisu 62

ultimate Bolognese 81

yemista with easy tzatziki 156

Y

yemista with easy tzatziki 156

yoghurt: chicken tikka masala 68

coconut chutney 86

easy tzatziki 156

mint yoghurt 138, 162

tahini yoghurt 146–7

Z

za'atar: tomato and pomegranate za'atar salad 208

zippy dippy 122

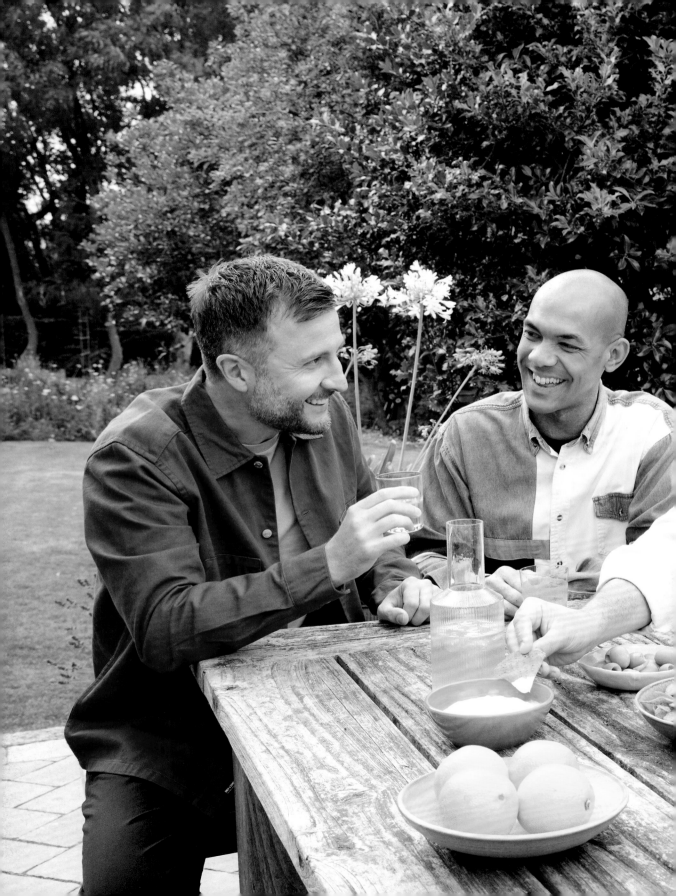

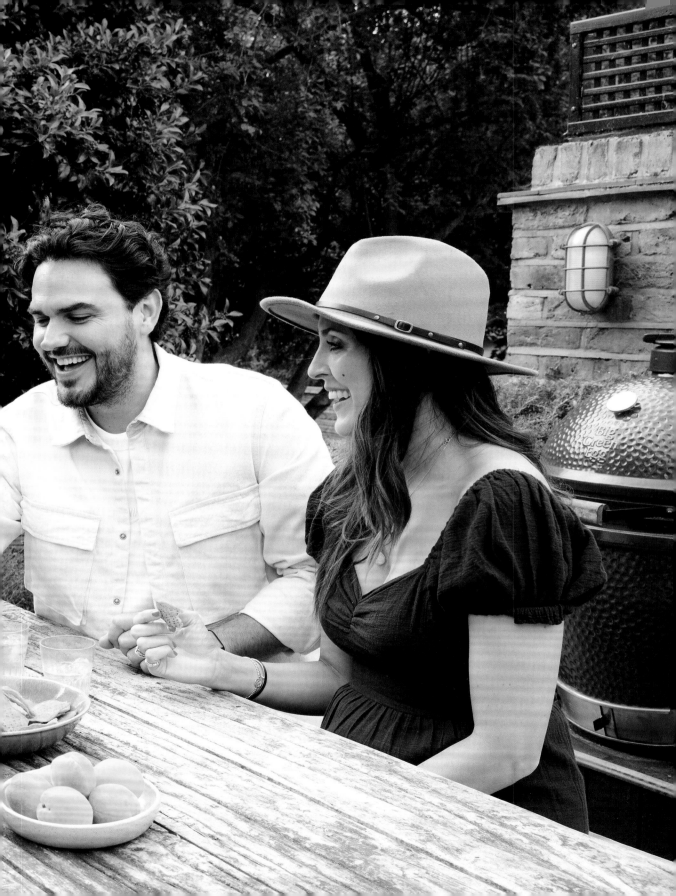

CONVERSION CHARTS

LIQUID MEASURES

Metric	Imperial
1.25ml	¼ tsp
2.5ml	½ tsp
5ml	1 tsp
15ml	1 tbsp
30ml	1fl oz (2 tbsp)
50ml	2fl oz
75ml	3fl oz
100ml	3½fl oz
125ml	4fl oz
150ml	5fl oz (¼ UK pint)
175ml	6fl oz
200ml	7fl oz
250ml	8fl oz
275ml	9fl oz
300ml	10fl oz (½ Imperial pint)
325ml	11fl oz
350ml	12fl oz
375ml	13fl oz
400ml	14fl oz
450ml	15fl oz (¾ pint)
475ml	16fl oz (1 US pint)
500ml	18fl oz
600ml	20fl oz (1 UK pint)
700ml	1¼ pints (25 fl oz)
850ml	1½ pints (30 fl oz)
1 litre	1¾ pints (35 fl oz)
1.2 litres	2 pints (40 fl oz)
1.3 litres	2¼ pints
1.4 litres	2½ pints
1.75 litres	3 pints
2 litres	3½ pints
3 litres	5 pints

SPOONS

1 tsp	5ml
1 dsp	10ml
1 tbsp (3 tsp)	15ml

DRY WEIGHTS

Metric	Imperial
10g	¼oz
15g	½oz
20g	¾oz
25g	1oz
40g	1½oz
50g	2oz
60g	2¼oz
70g	2¾oz
75g	3oz
100g	3½oz
115g	4oz
125g	4½oz
140g	4¾oz
150g	5oz
160g	5½oz
175g	6oz
200g	7oz
225g	8oz
250g	9oz
275g	9½oz
300g	11oz
350g	12oz
375g	13oz
400g	14oz
425g	15oz
450g	16oz (1lb)
500g (0.5kg)	1lb 2oz
550g	1¼lb
600g	1lb 5oz
675g	1½lb
725g	1lb 10oz
800g	1¾lb
850g	1lb 14oz
900g	2lb
1kg	2¼lb
1.1kg	2½lb
1.25kg	2¾lb
1.3kg	3lb
1.5kg	3¼lb
1.6kg	3½lb
1.8kg	4lb
2kg	4½lb

ACKNOWLEDGEMENTS

Our creative team, who got this one-of-a-kind book over the line: Lizzie Mayson for the marvellous food photography • Nicky Johnston for the lovely photos of us and our friends • Ellie Mulligan for the expert food styling • Louie Waller for the excellent prop styling • Em-J for the artistic and vegan-friendly makeup • Alexis Knox for the cracking clobber • Jack from Neville and Issey from Larry King for the super fresh trims

Our publishing team, for producing our best book yet: Nira Begum • Lisa Milton, thanks so much for being so forward thinking and letting us write this book • Charlie Redmayne for your continued support • Lucy Sykes-Thompson for the beautiful book design • Laura Nickoll for your razor-sharp copy-editing skills • Georgina Green for managing the sales of this book so professionally • Joanna Rose, Dawn Burnett, Lucy Richardson, Komal Patel and Sian Baldwin for generating so much wonderful exposure • Lizzie Mayson for letting us use your wonderful studio • Bev James and team, thanks for everything

TEAM BOSH! for all your hard work: Nat, Anna, Lily, Guy, Tom, Elior, Joe, Nicole, Yoon, Gabrielė, Louise, Charlie, Sepps, Cat, Emily, Laila – you're all legends and we're lucky to work with you • David and Gabby at Dundas – your integrity and great work helps us all make better food choices • Our food team, for ensuring everyone who uses this book experiences 100% deliciousness • Lily Harris, Luke Robinson, Emily Dobbs, Elena Silcock and Sareta Puri: you all did SUCH a great job – plants have never tasted so meaty! • Everyone at Fiddes Payne, Finsbury, Oscar Mayer, IG Design and Baxters – thanks for helping us put more plants on plates

Geoff, Paul, Mark, Steff, Sir Crispin, David, Frank, Stephen, Liz, Mark, Guy, Tomas, Jerome, Michael, Ekow, Regine, Clive, Stephen, Rupert, Sarah, Sean, Alex, Anna – thanks for believing in BOSH! It's great to have you all on the journey with us!

Henry's people: EmJ, Berry and Chippy • Jane and Mark • Alice, Graham and little baby James • Chris, Paul and Tom Williams • Sukey, Nick, Gus and Arthur • Bruce, thinking of you x • Claire, Nick and Xander • Alison and Curtis • John Dodd, Zoe and Stanley • Davey P, Ben and Rosie

Ian's people: Sarah • Mum, Dad, Frances, Stew and Phoebe • Paul, Sue, Nick, Lesley and Alexander, Sean and Mills, Alex and Meg, Jamie and Milly, Mikey • Carolyn, Edward and Philip • Robin and Suzie • Josephine, Katie, Mike and Kev • Steve, Shirley, Lynsey and Kerry

Our good buds: Alex, Tara and Cillian • Kweku, Angie and Akaiya • Tom, Emilie, Alex and Ruby • Darren and Danielle • Anna, Beth and Rupert • Mutty • Nat, Khairan, Lennox, Ziyah and Imani • Marcus, Ellie, Jasper, Caspian, Nia and Sylvan • Ekow, Claire, Hugo and Xander • Zulf, Farhana, Ayza, Ayla and Rumi • Addison, Claire, Lola Grace, August and Stanley • Maso, Bex, Finn and Piper • Tom, Stef, Romy and Essie • CB and Nikita • Luke • Nish and Rachel • Martha, Duncan, Ernie and Morris • Josh, Charlotte, Leo, Uma and Ocho • Tim, Susie, Wren and Ember • Alex Farbz, Cat, Freddie and Samuel • Akash and Dilshad • Nick, Ruth and Finn • Janey and Jack • Joe, Ted and the fam • Louis • Leslie • Joel, Liana, Miles and bump

Everyone who works in and around the plant-based food space, you inspire us – thank you for all you do • Thanks to all the plant-based meat, fish and protein brands for pushing the world forward, innovating, and making ethical, sustainable food choices available for everyone. You all made this book possible • Massive thanks to everyone who follows us on social media – every like, share and comment ensures our plant-based food videos are seen by millions

Most importantly, THANK YOU! Thank you so much for buying this book – we hope you find your new favourite meal in these pages.

For more plant-based recipes and inspiration, head to www.bosh.tv